Heart
Attack

Cephas

Thank you for sharing your incredible gift of music with us at the launch! God must have shared the blueprint from King David in his creation of you; surely a man after his heart — humble, generous of spirit, a poet & musician and dashing!;S

May your life be filled with radiant light. Live inspired

Heart Attack

Finding hope, joy and inspiration through adversity

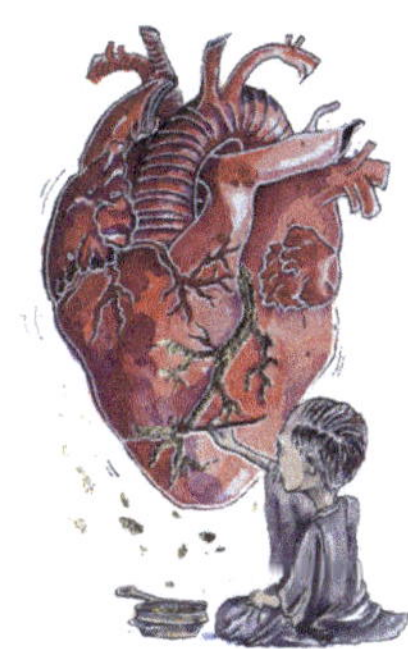

WRITTEN AND ILLUSTRATED BY

Jeff Schmidt

Dedicated to

my family and friends – the people who constantly remind me that light shines brightest in the darkest spaces.

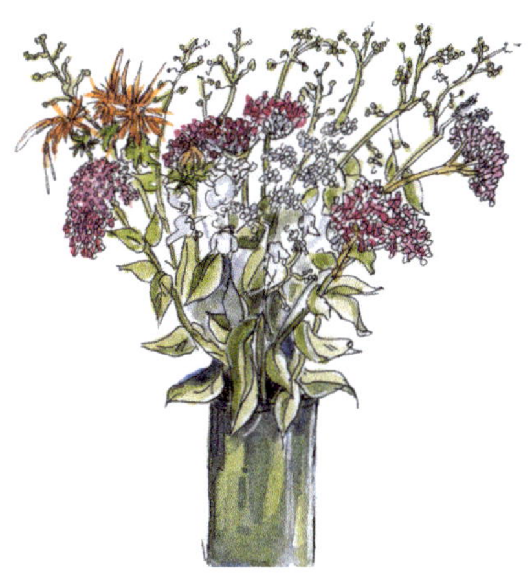

Published under licence by Brown Dog Books and The Self-Publishing Partnership Ltd, 10b Greenway Farm, Bath Rd,
Wick, nr. Bath BS30 5RL

www.selfpublishingpartnership.co.uk

ISBN printed book: 978-1-83952-498-1
ISBN e-book: 978-1-83952-499-8

Edited by Di Bach and Janet Clark
Cover design and illustrations by Jeff Schmidt
Internal layout by Andrew Easton

Printed and bound in the UK

This book is printed on FSC certified paper

DOWNLOAD THE AUDIOBOOK FREE!

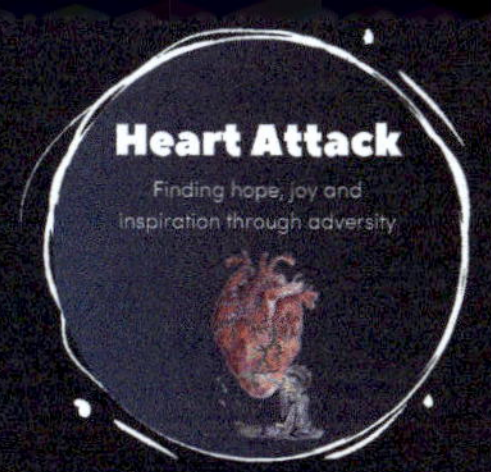

READ THIS FIRST

Thank you for purchasing 'Heart Attack- Finding hope, joy and inspiration through adversity'.

Knowing that audiobooks can make a story feel more like a warm conversation with an old friend than an impartial account from a stranger, I have recorded the audio version for you as a gift.

Visit the following page or scan the QR code to access the book free of charge.

https://subscribepage.io/Audiobook

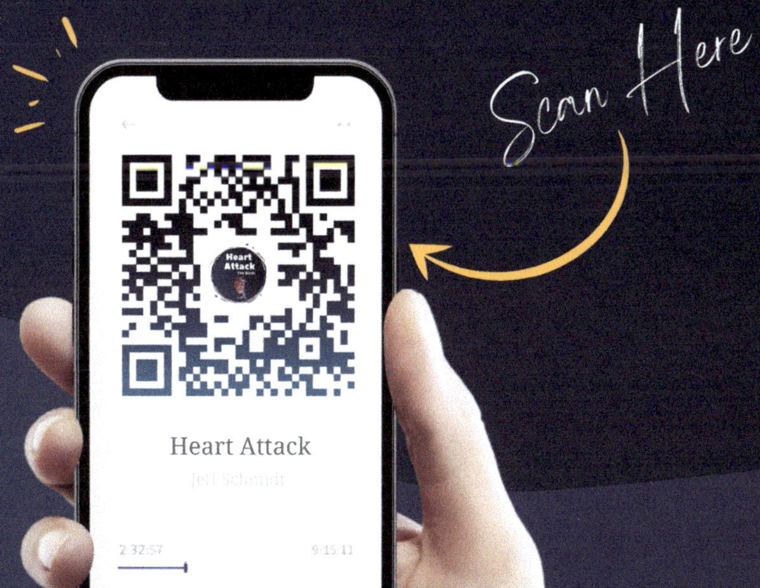

FOREWORD
(A word from the heart)

This is my first foreword. I searched on Google 'how to write a foreword'. It boils down to three Cs: the content of the book; your connection with the author; and what would compel someone to read the book. It seemed simple enough.

But not for this book. If you've started reading at the foreword, pause. Now, flick through the pages. Allow those interdigitating illustrations to play visual havoc with your retina. This is a book written by an extraordinary middle-aged man called Jeff, whose life is irretrievably shattered by a rapid-fire succession of heart attacks; this book has pictures, also drawn by Jeff. Because when the indescribably awful happens to us, and the impact weighs heavy on our loved ones, words are not enough. This is a courageous life story that speaks as much to the questing intellect of the mind as it does to the raw vulnerability of the heart.

"There is perhaps nothing we modern people need more than to be genuinely shaken up. Where life is firm, we need to know its firmness; and where it is unstable and uncertain and has no basis, no foundation, we need to know this too and to endure it." [Alfred Delf]

Before the cardiac event, Jeff was living a life stretched taut between the self-persuaded invincibility of youth and the self-propelled ambitions of middle age. I should say, 'lived'. Past tense.

What happened that evening, when the heart attack knocked on the door of Jeff's life, and he unwittingly opened that door, revealed at least three of his core motivations for living life fully. The first, approach adversity as you would an unexpected friend rather than an unwelcome intrusion. The second, let your intrepid quest for success be in the things of life that truly matter. The third, deep relationships usher the liminal luminosity of hope into life's darkest corners.

I thought that writing a foreword would be fiendishly hard. Doubly so when the author is a dear friend. It is impossible to avoid carrying even a nebulous sense of responsibility for the reader's response. I needn't have worried. Jeff writes the way he speaks, the way he lives, and the way he inspires. He is less a man defined by what he does or says, as much as a man who lives out fiercely, faithfully and fearlessly the process of 'becoming'. And in this book, it is this invitation that he extends to you, the reader.

There is much to appreciate in this book. Please don't read it simply for that reason. Read Jeff's story prepared, poised even, to find your own story in these pages, to be challenged, and to be changed, from the heart.

Dr Esther Chew

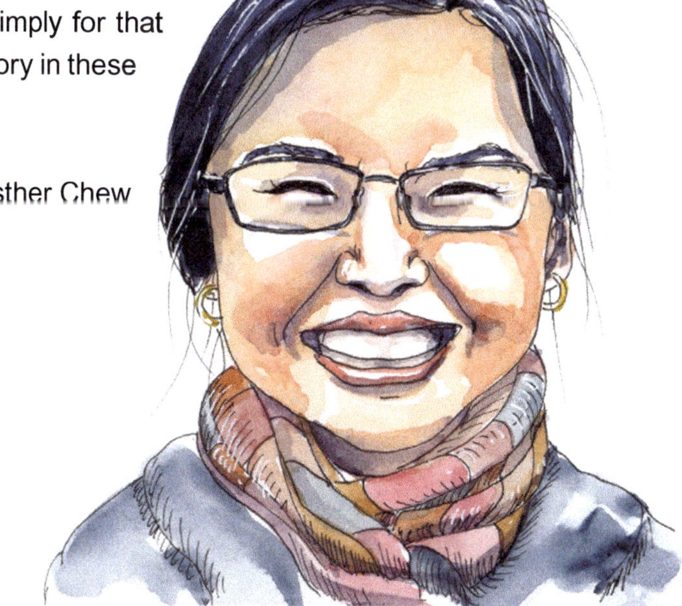

Trauma

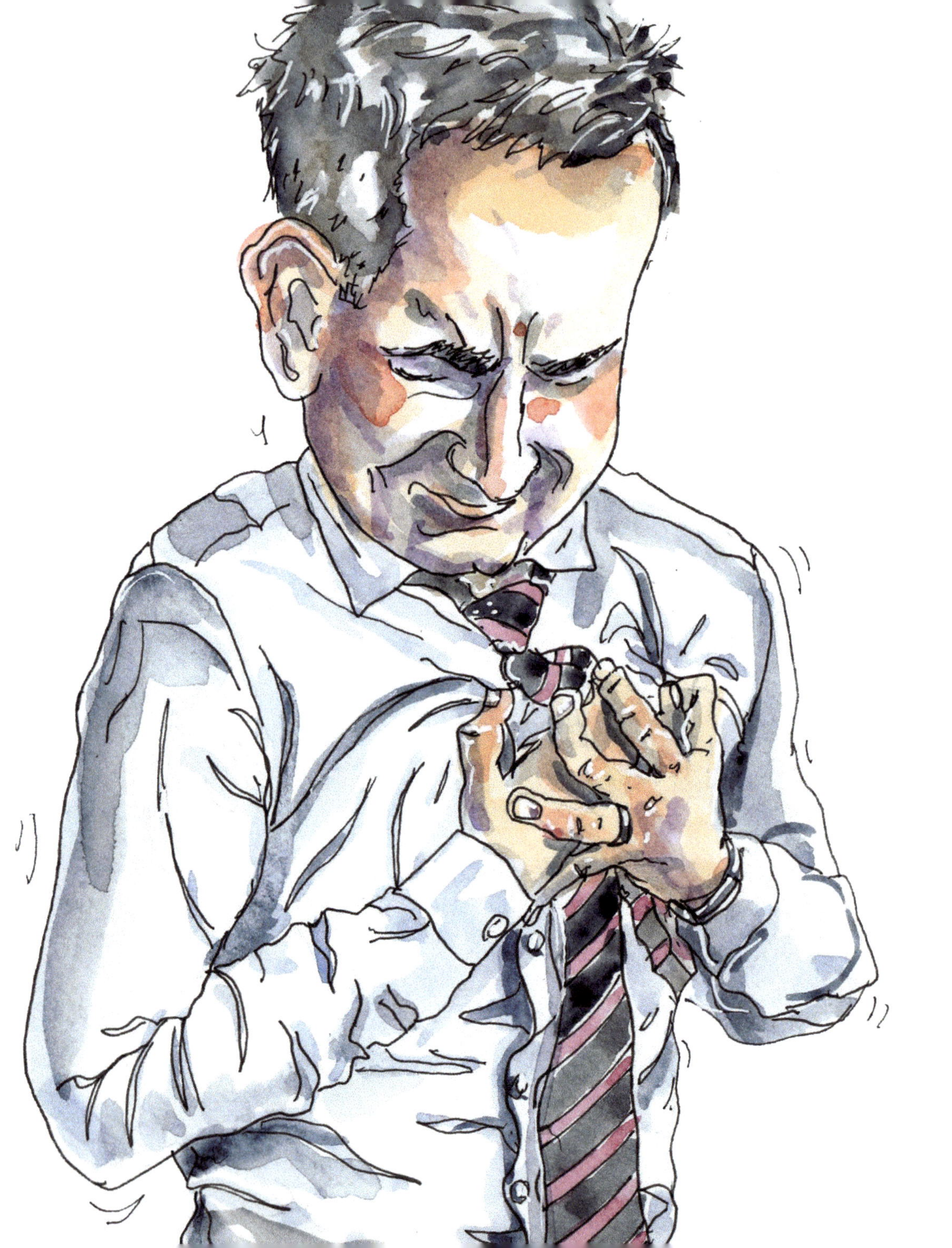

BLEEP, BLEEP, BLEEP

THAT IS THE SOUND of life, and it is the sound of a hospital. A hospital is a world unlike any other. Within it there is a constant flow of people, all people, regardless of clan or creed, status or influence. They gather for a united purpose, to maintain life. At the most basic level, people are all just an intricate amalgamation of cells, delicately knitted together to enable movement, growth and interaction. As wonderful as it is, this design is imperfect (increasingly so as we age) and we are often unaware of its gift until it crashes.

I crashed. Unexpectedly. My perceived superpowers ran out, mortal kryptonite finally seizing its opportunity to take control.

And so, I found myself in hospital. In an instant, or rather a strained, chest-crushing, arm-aching, jaw-clenching series of 'attacks', I was removed from the life I knew, as a (relatively) healthy overambitious 40-something professional and plunged into a strange new world. The journey was, and continues to be, profound. There have been many bleeps, groans and characters, certainly much bustling but, most significantly, there has been change.

At my side, a ubiquitous 0.1mm pen and a trusty watercolour pan, candidly recording my recovery – the joy, the pain, the unexpected and the revelation.

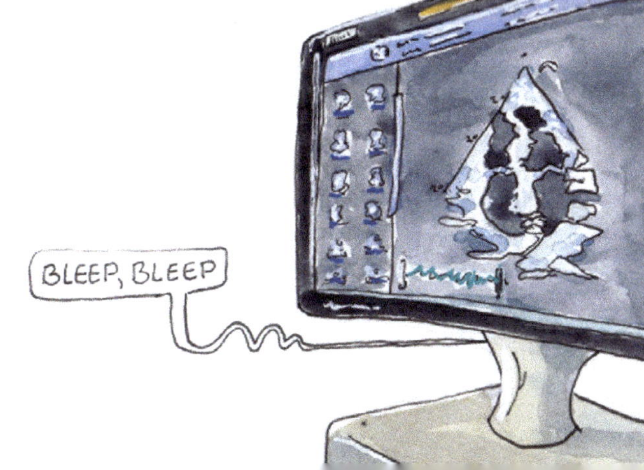

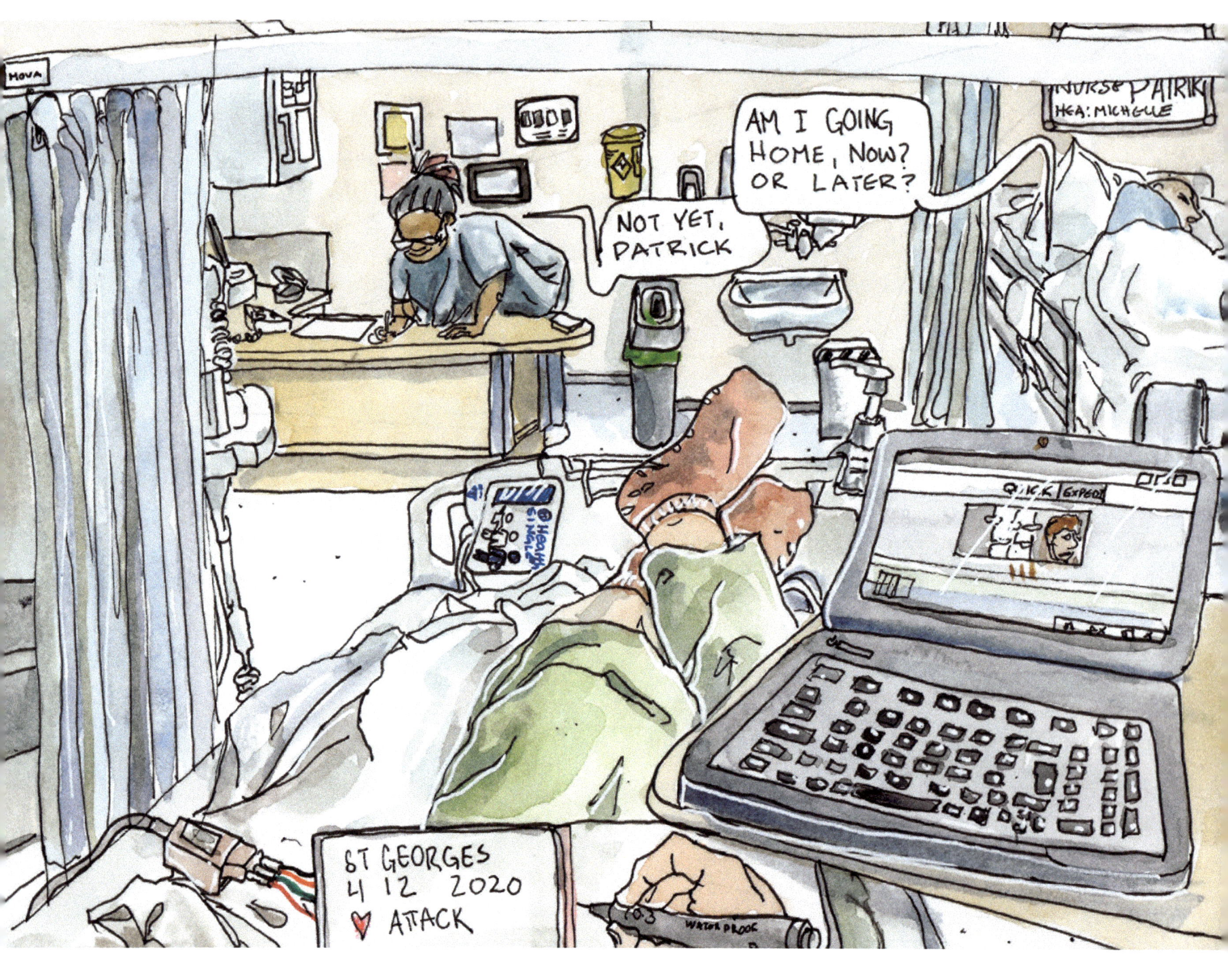

MOVA
NURSE PATRIK
HEA: MICHELLE
AM I GOING HOME, NOW? OR LATER?
NOT YET, PATRICK
QUICK EXPOSE
ST GEORGES
4 12 2020
ATTACK
WATERPROOF

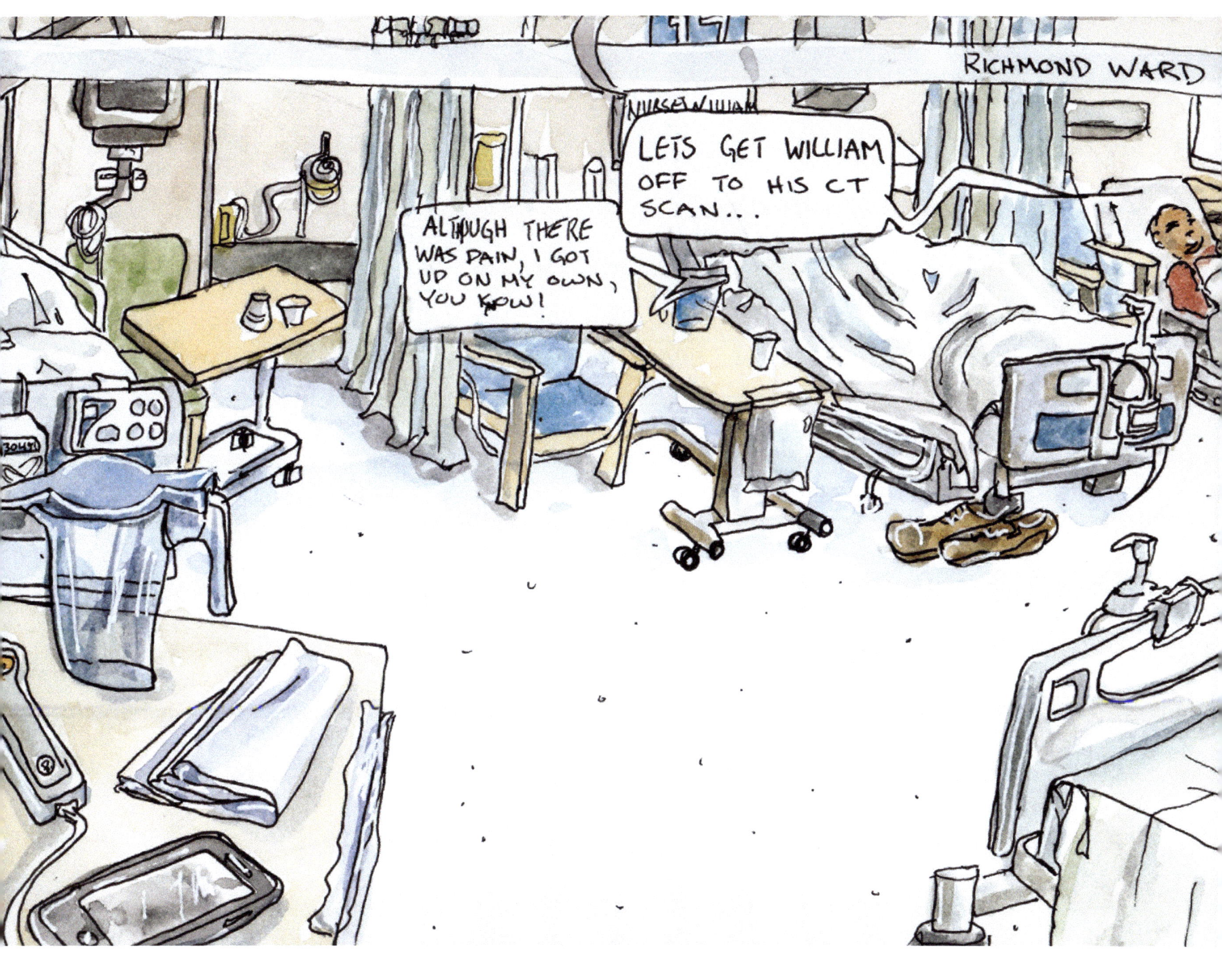
RICHMOND WARD
NURSE WILLIAM
LETS GET WILLIAM OFF TO HIS CT SCAN...
ALTHOUGH THERE WAS PAIN, I GOT UP ON MY OWN, YOU KNOW!

MATTERS OF THE HEART

WHEN YOU TAMPER with matters of the heart, metaphorical or otherwise, it is all-consuming – whether falling in (or out) of love, being thrust into imminent danger, celebrating triumphantly or meddling with something you hold dear. I have seen and felt the impact of these events at various times throughout my life. For instance, at the tender age of 14, I remember experiencing my first palpable crush with its flurry of torturous emotions. At the crescendo of this newly formed 'relationship', I had mustered up all my courage and poured out my heart to the beautiful young vixen behind the school baseball bleachers only to be rejected with a pretentious laugh that echoed endlessly in my head (and heart) for weeks. Still, at 46, I recoil at the thought of that moment. But regardless of whether it is heartbreak or love, the thrill of victoriously raising a trophy or coming face-to-face with death, they all have a deep impact. And they all insist that you stop and take stock of your life.

'That' evening, the one that irreversibly shook up my life, Thursday 3 December, I found myself staring eternity squarely in the face. I had returned home with my two girls. It had been a stressful day capped by a suitably heated, hard-hitting quarrel that left me trembling. I would not generally consider my life stressful, and yet I know that I run at a pretty high-octane pace. But that's OK, because, despite warnings from others, I am, or believed I was, bulletproof. I wore my intensity like a shiny badge of honour. On that evening, however, the engine said *'no more'*; you can't drive even the most brilliantly engineered sports cars at 5000 RPM indefinitely. It took my mum, who spotted me bent over, clutching my chest, rubbing my arms on FaceTime and my daughter's subsequent fear-filled plea to get help for me to make the medical call. Reluctantly, in a haze of pain, I did make the call. In minutes an ambulance was there. Pride masking the danger, I couldn't help but feel that all this commotion was quite unnecessary. The seasoned paramedics quickly assessed my traumatised frame, blood pressure surging through my veins like a blocked firehose. They looked me straight in the eyes, piercing my vanity, and said, "We are taking you to hospital. Now." These two burly, tattoo-laden men not only had the expertise to see what was physically happening but the gift to see much deeper, to the matters of the heart.

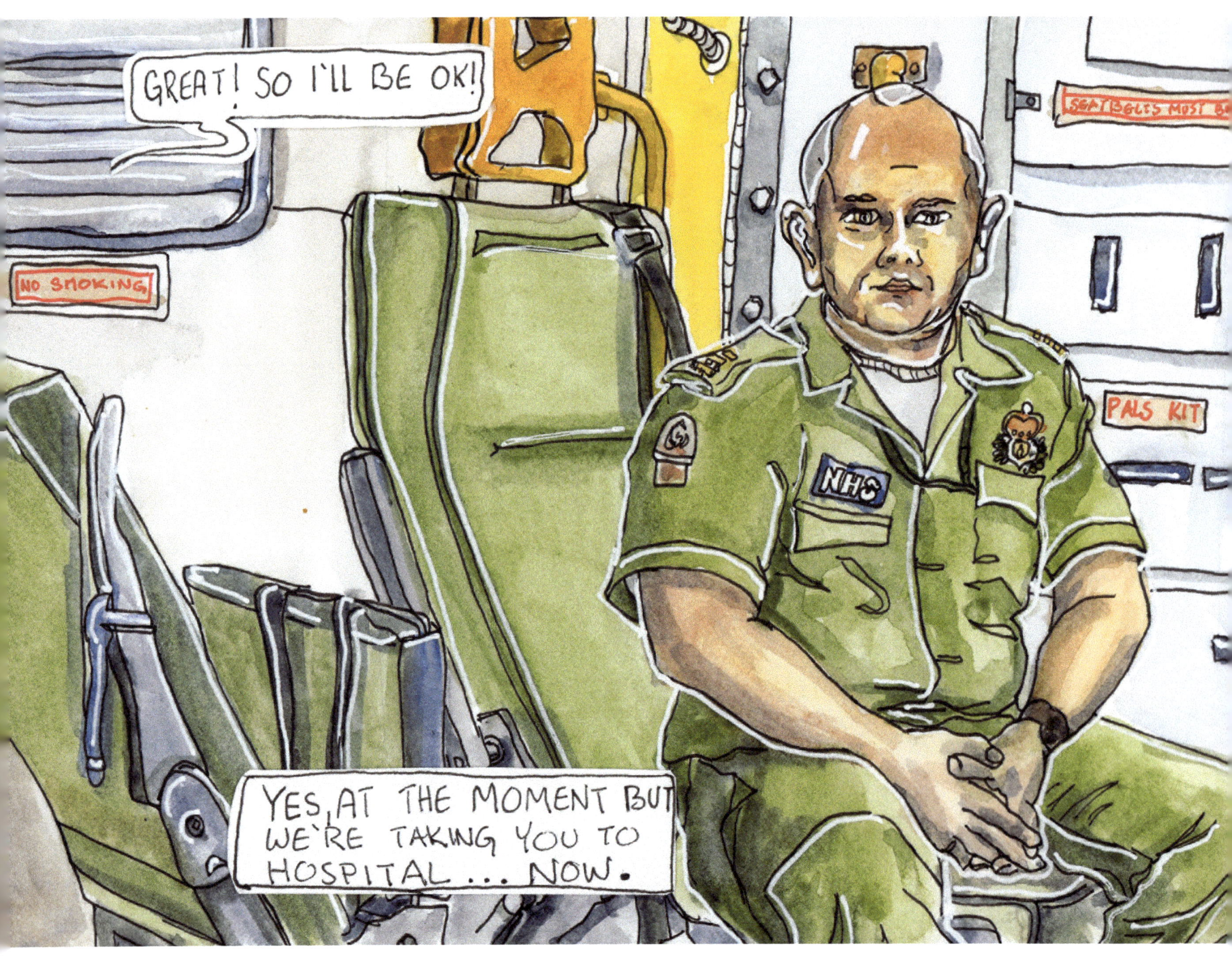

GREAT! SO I'LL BE OK!
NO SMOKING
SEATBELTS MUST
PALS KIT
NHS
YES, AT THE MOMENT BUT WE'RE TAKING YOU TO HOSPITAL ... NOW.

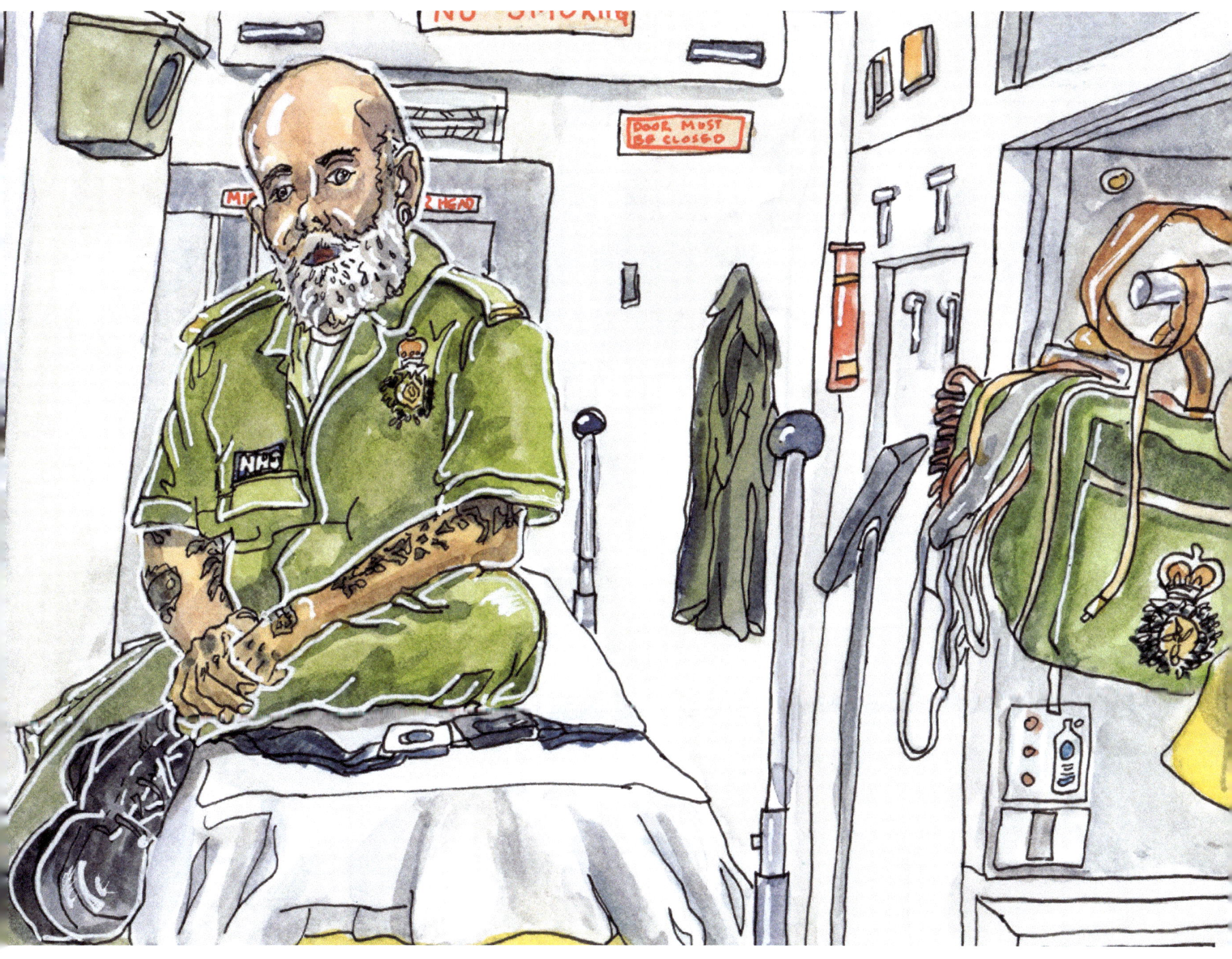

NO SMOKING
DOOR MUST BE CLOSED
NHS

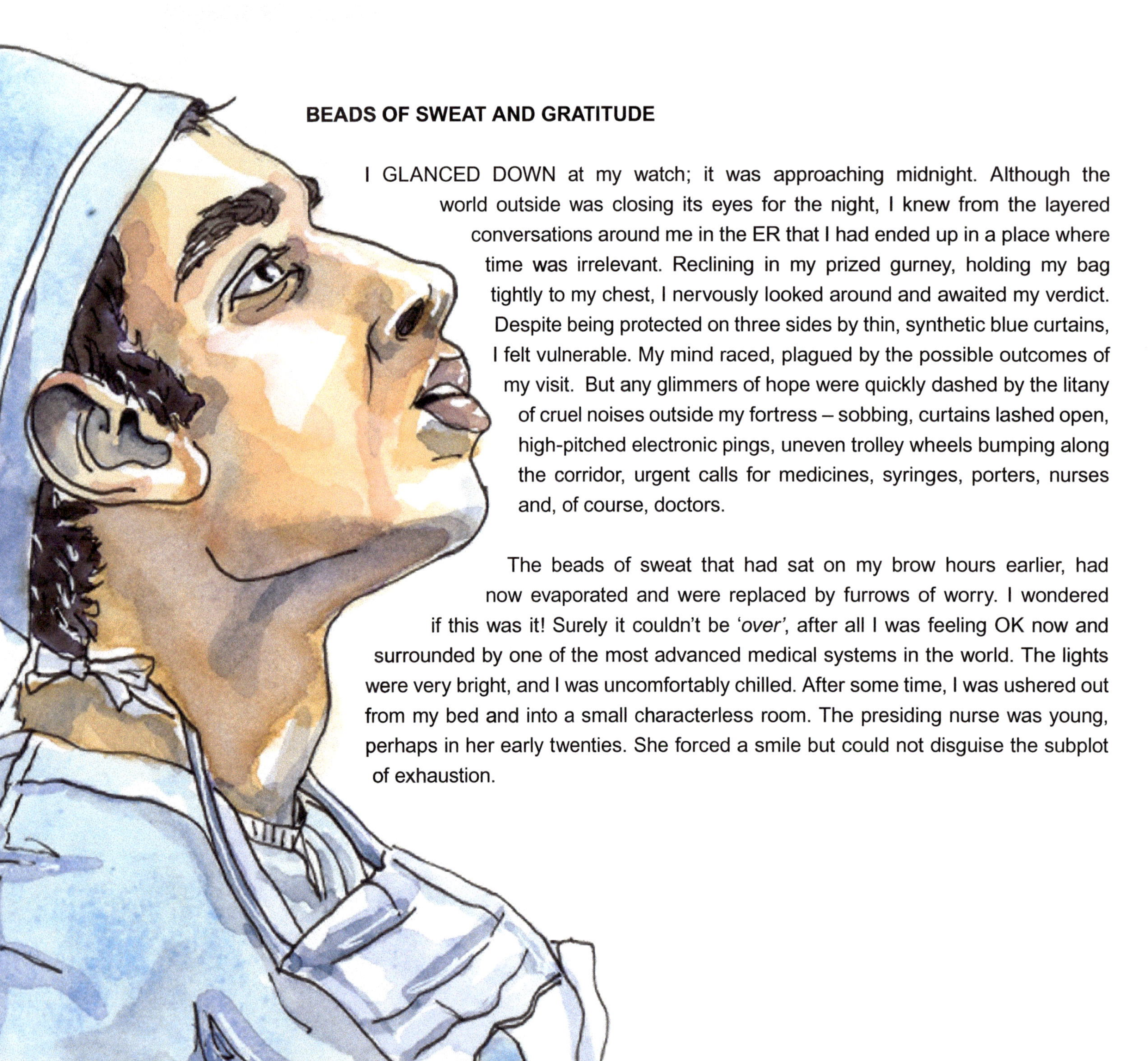

BEADS OF SWEAT AND GRATITUDE

I GLANCED DOWN at my watch; it was approaching midnight. Although the world outside was closing its eyes for the night, I knew from the layered conversations around me in the ER that I had ended up in a place where time was irrelevant. Reclining in my prized gurney, holding my bag tightly to my chest, I nervously looked around and awaited my verdict. Despite being protected on three sides by thin, synthetic blue curtains, I felt vulnerable. My mind raced, plagued by the possible outcomes of my visit. But any glimmers of hope were quickly dashed by the litany of cruel noises outside my fortress – sobbing, curtains lashed open, high-pitched electronic pings, uneven trolley wheels bumping along the corridor, urgent calls for medicines, syringes, porters, nurses and, of course, doctors.

The beads of sweat that had sat on my brow hours earlier, had now evaporated and were replaced by furrows of worry. I wondered if this was it! Surely it couldn't be *'over'*, after all I was feeling OK now and surrounded by one of the most advanced medical systems in the world. The lights were very bright, and I was uncomfortably chilled. After some time, I was ushered out from my bed and into a small characterless room. The presiding nurse was young, perhaps in her early twenties. She forced a smile but could not disguise the subplot of exhaustion.

"The doctor will be with you shortly," she murmured in a diluted Caribbean accent. She disappeared around the corner, and I could hear her flicking through the papers on her clipboard. I waited. More thinking time. "Maybe it won't be so bad," I thought to myself, "I'm sure it won't be that bad."

The resident doctor arrived. I noted a few beads of sweat pocking his forehead. Evidently, I was not the only one with a dollop of stress on his plate that evening. He dropped to his chair and pushed his wire-rimmed spectacles up the bridge of his nose revealing the redness around his eyes. He asked me for the usual catalogue of credentials: name, birthdate and address.

"Well, Mr Schmidt, the results are in," he said matter-of-factly. "You have had a heart attack, likely a series of heart attacks."

Shock. I struggled to understand how that was possible. My mind swirled.

Then, as I stared at the blank wall in that lonely cubicle, an unexpected revelation crept in to make space in the melee of emotions. Hollow memories of a little Hans Christian Andersen quote from years earlier rumbled deep within, "The whole world is a series of miracles ... but we are so used to them we call them ordinary things." Almost nothing amazes us anymore. We grow up, acclimatise to the world and take most things for granted. But in that moment, there in front of me, was a man, an extraordinary man who had given years of his life pursuing a calling so that he might help others. On this day he helped me! That is amazing!

There in that room, awe regained its rightful place from the tyranny of self-pity. I am learning that you can find so much goodness in the most unlikely circumstances.

THERE'S THIS COMEDY ABOUT THESE 3 GUYS ...

SOMETIMES it is hard to find that silver lining in life, and yet, blessings are often there, all around us.

As I laid in my Swiss Army knife of a hospital bed (they can do the most incredible things!), I observed the undulating dynamics of the hospital ward. There were some really sick people – knocking on death's door kind of sick – complete with groans, grunts and other strange bodily noises. Others were old, some grumpy and demanding, while others waited patiently, almost lost in a trance of hopelessness. A select few extraordinary individuals exuded a spirit of gratefulness in all things, even in the smallest things, a warm passing smile or a nod to one's presence. In the background was COVID, the looming plague, which did little to help morale. Distances were kept, visitors could not infiltrate the firmly locked doors and masks served as a constant reminder of the many imposed restrictions. In amongst it all, the nurses buzzed around, despite their own afflictions, attending to the endless needs of their patients.

Sitting there, with a broken heart, preparing to hunker down for the sake of self-preservation, I heard a voice. Through the busyness and despair arose an upbeat chortle, a slice of goodness. Words that, not only in their content but by their very nature, seemed to lift the atmosphere of the room.

"You can't win them all, Michelle!" I turned to see a nurse respond to a patient with an unaided smile. Then he punctuated the comment with a happy wink and a sincere, "Thank you."

It was the voice of David. An accomplished man, a judge, with none of the trappings that traditionally consume those with power. He would grow to become a lifeline, a partner in crime, an amigo with whom I was not merely to survive, but thrive. And naturally these kinds of people draw others in with their irresistible gravity. So after day two, Mark had also joined the merry band and then there was three. Journeying together, with levity and authenticity, bumped from one ward to another, through procedures and fears, we shared a deep sense of kinship.

At one point, after having weathered a few days in the trenches together, Mark mused, "There's this comedy from the 70s about these three guys who were all stuck in hospital together for weeks on end, you never quite knew why they were there ... but it worked!" I suppose that's the nub of it. In hospital you are torn from the things you know, plunged into the unpredictable, left to forge a life with a random assortment of companions, and, if you are lucky, it works.

Then again, maybe it's not luck, but rather the silver lining waiting to be discovered.

*David and Mark, thank you for the moments of hilarity and connection, I am a richer man for it.

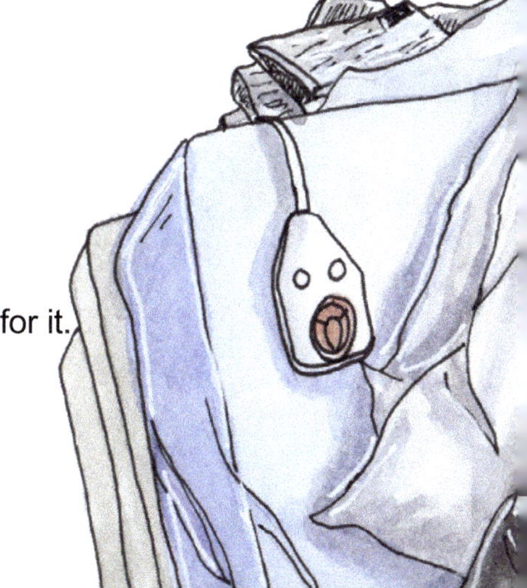

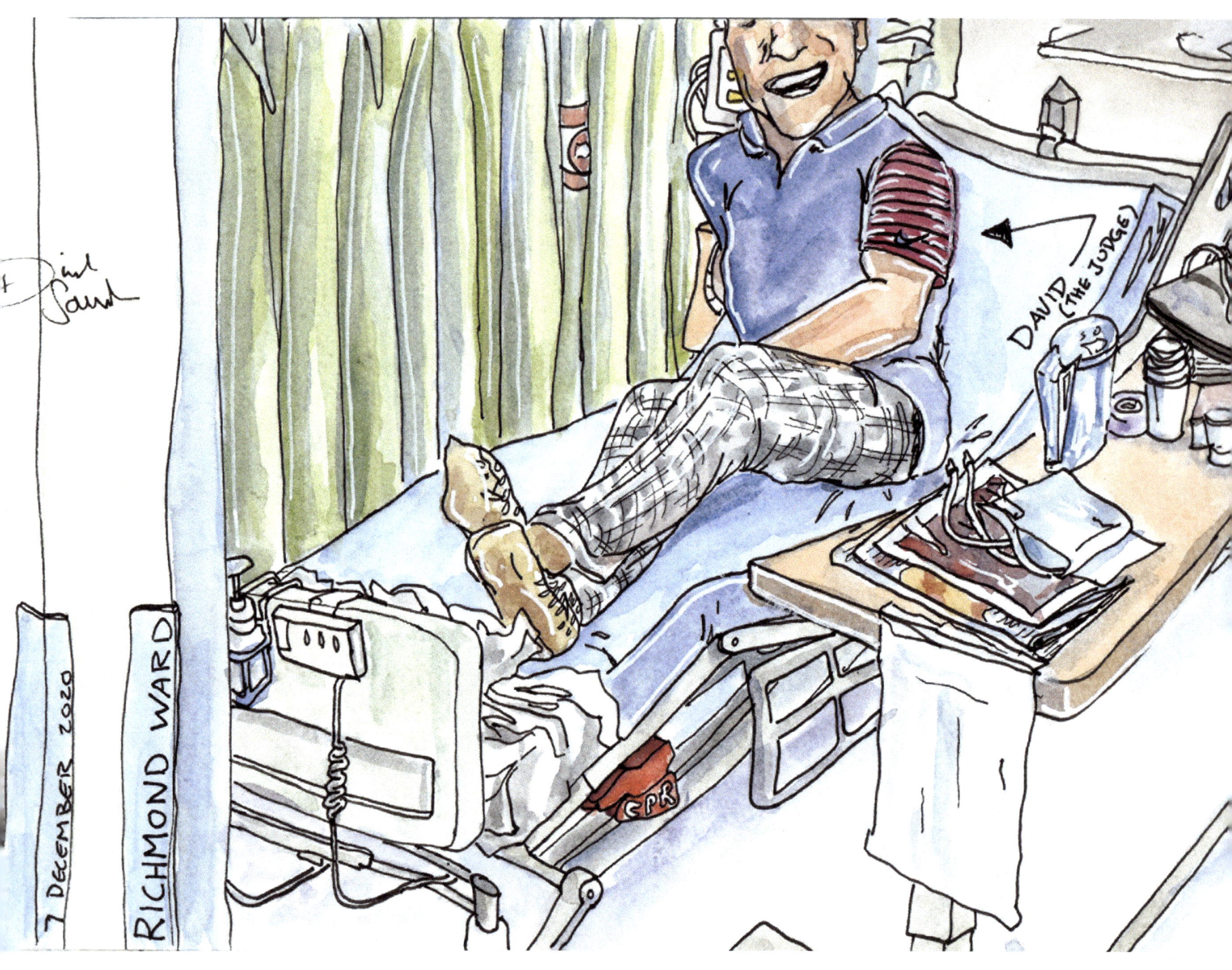

DAVID (THE JUDGE)
CPR
RICHMOND WARD
7 DECEMBER 2020

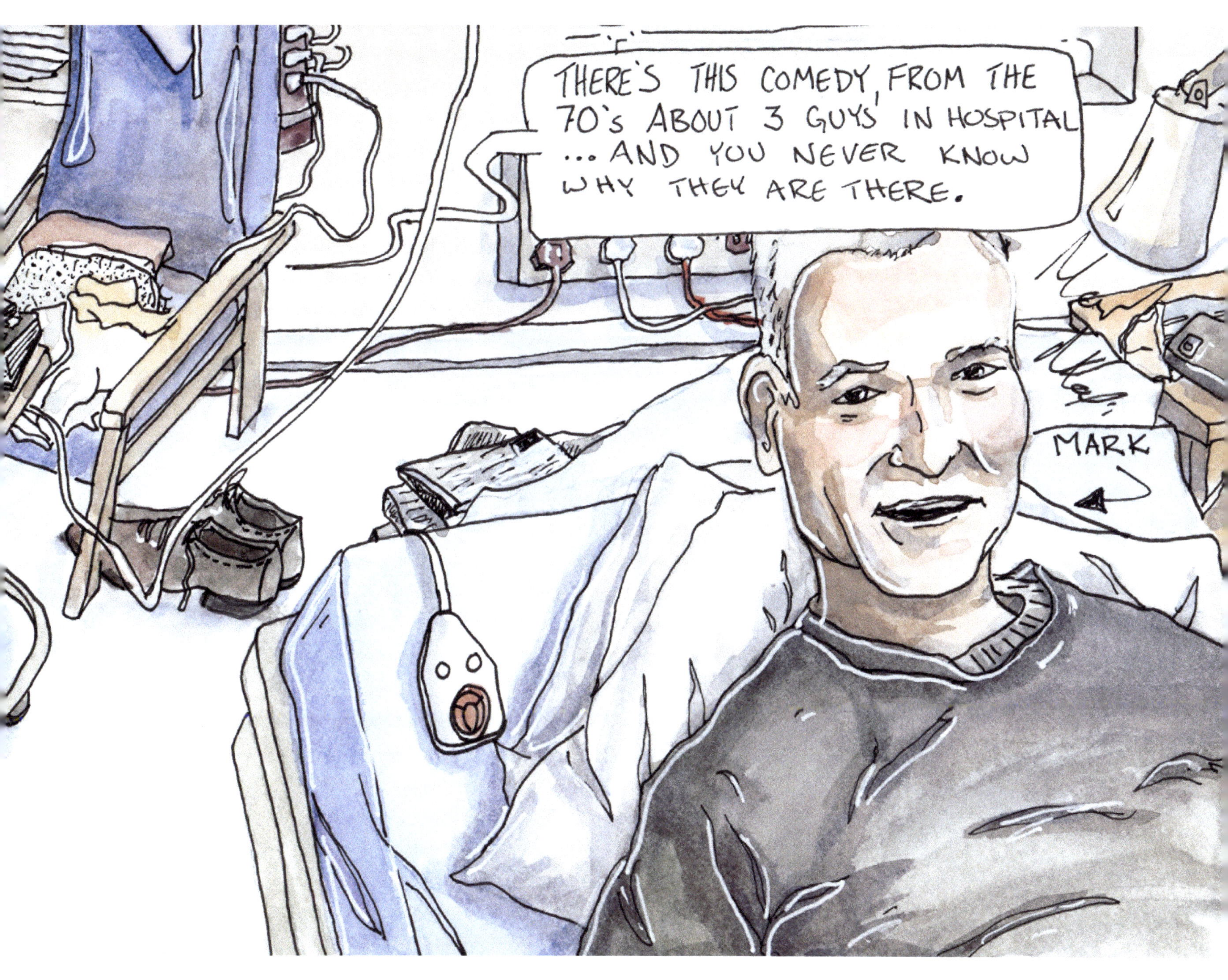

THERE'S THIS COMEDY, FROM THE 70's ABOUT 3 GUYS' IN HOSPITAL ...AND YOU NEVER KNOW WHY THEY ARE THERE.
MARK

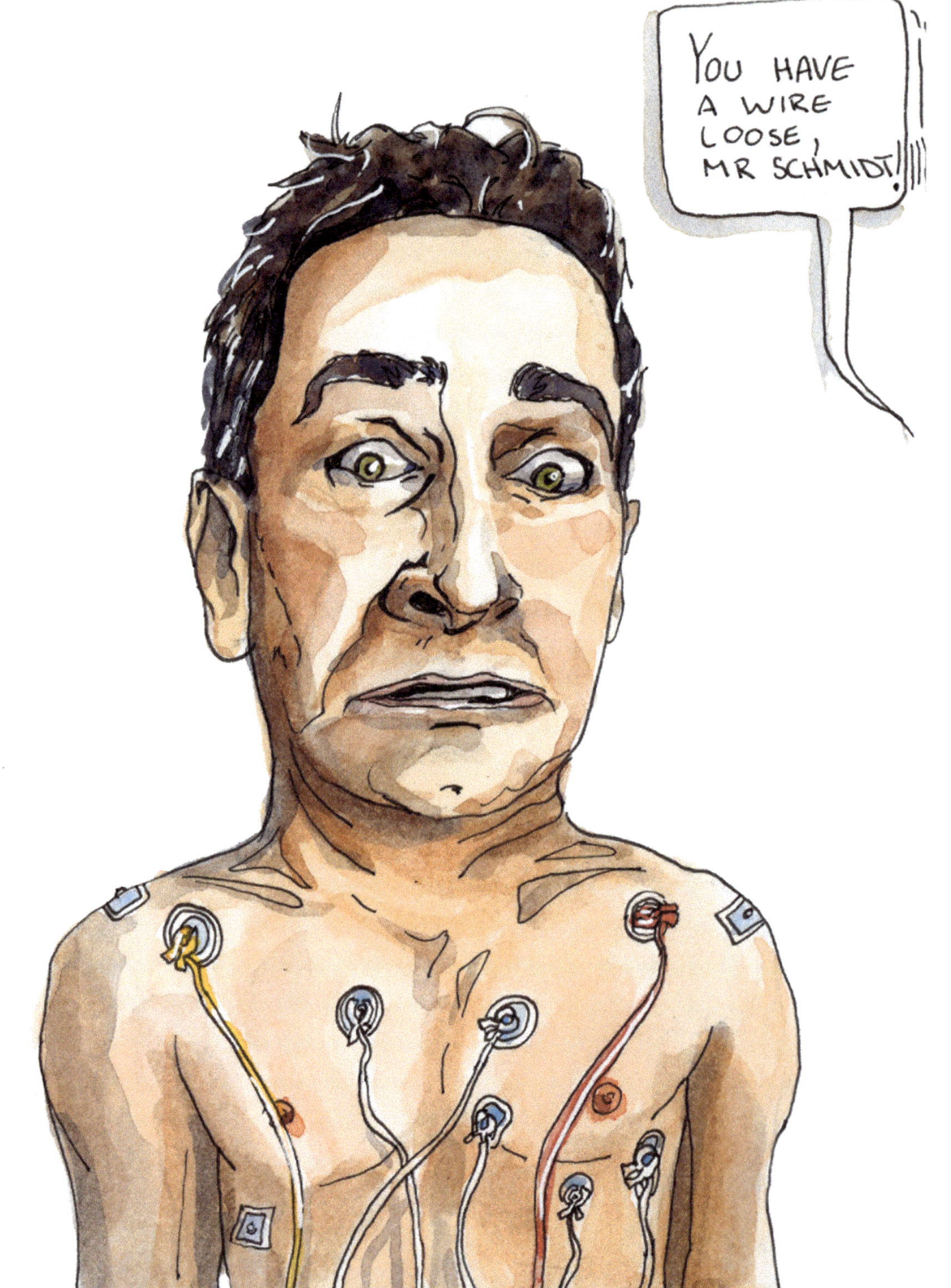

YOU HAVE
A WIRE
LOOSE,
MR SCHMIDT!

WIRED

"MR SCHMIDT. WAKE UP! Wake up! It seems you have a wire loose. Our monitors are warning us that something is wrong!"

Shaken awake, in the wee hours of the morning, there was a frantic and continuous beeping beside my head. My heartrate surged. Fear instantly took hold. A nurse leaned over to check my leads, a few wiggles and a sigh, "Ah, there it is, Mr Schmidt," she said in a hushed voice, "that should bring us back to normal." Sure enough, the machine responded with a delicate chorus of lines steadily dancing in time on the tiny monitor. Reassured, I drifted back off to sleep.

The day before had been unusual and significant. It had started routinely enough; the fluorescent bulbs of the ward unceremoniously flickering on at 6 a.m. sharp and the usual battery of tests – blood pressure, temperature, pulse and an ECG for good measure. Morning meds and breakfast were issued, then we waited for the doctors to do their rounds. On this day, one of our wardmates returned early from his operation, similar to the one we would all be undergoing, a 'fairly routine' angiogram and stent procedure. He gaily reported back to us that it was a success, not his first, nor his only medical issue but, on the whole, he was feeling fine and looking forward to getting back onto his feet.

His physio soon arrived to discuss mobility issues. They shared a few moments of humour and just as he had completed a few short steps, he remarked that he was feeling slightly dizzy. That's where the day turned. Within seconds, he dropped. Just like in Hollywood films, his monitor started to frantically bleep, then the bleeping turned to a single high-pitched squeal. Calls for help. Curtains were whipped shut. The alarm was raised, and medical staff flooded the room. Expertly directed by a doctor, people slid in and out of the cubicle. Terrible noises punctuated the atmosphere, exhumed from a lifeless body. CPR. More gut-wrenching noises. Defib ...

After what seemed like an eternity, and at least four minutes without a heartbeat, life was miraculously restored. Many of my fellow wardmates, those who could, had now left their beds and were nervously pacing the far end of the room. Their arms tightly crossed, and barely audible mumblings exposed what lay behind their deeply sombre expressions.

The medical staff, however, were extraordinary. Working with calm, clarity and symbiotic harmony they had brought our friend back to life. Looking across to his bed, he was fast asleep and safe – underscored by the steady ballet of lines rippling across his monitor. Once again, fully wired.

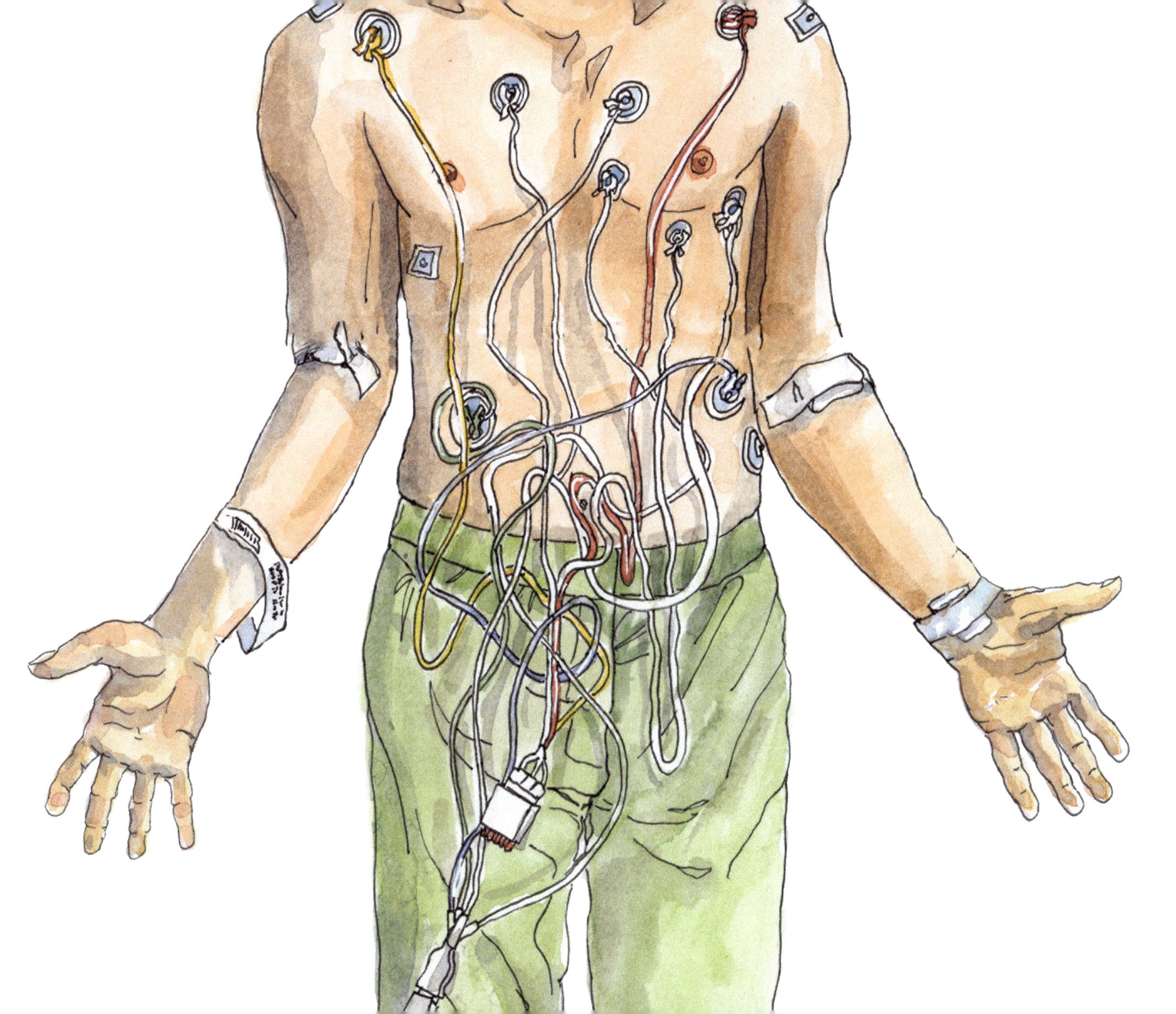

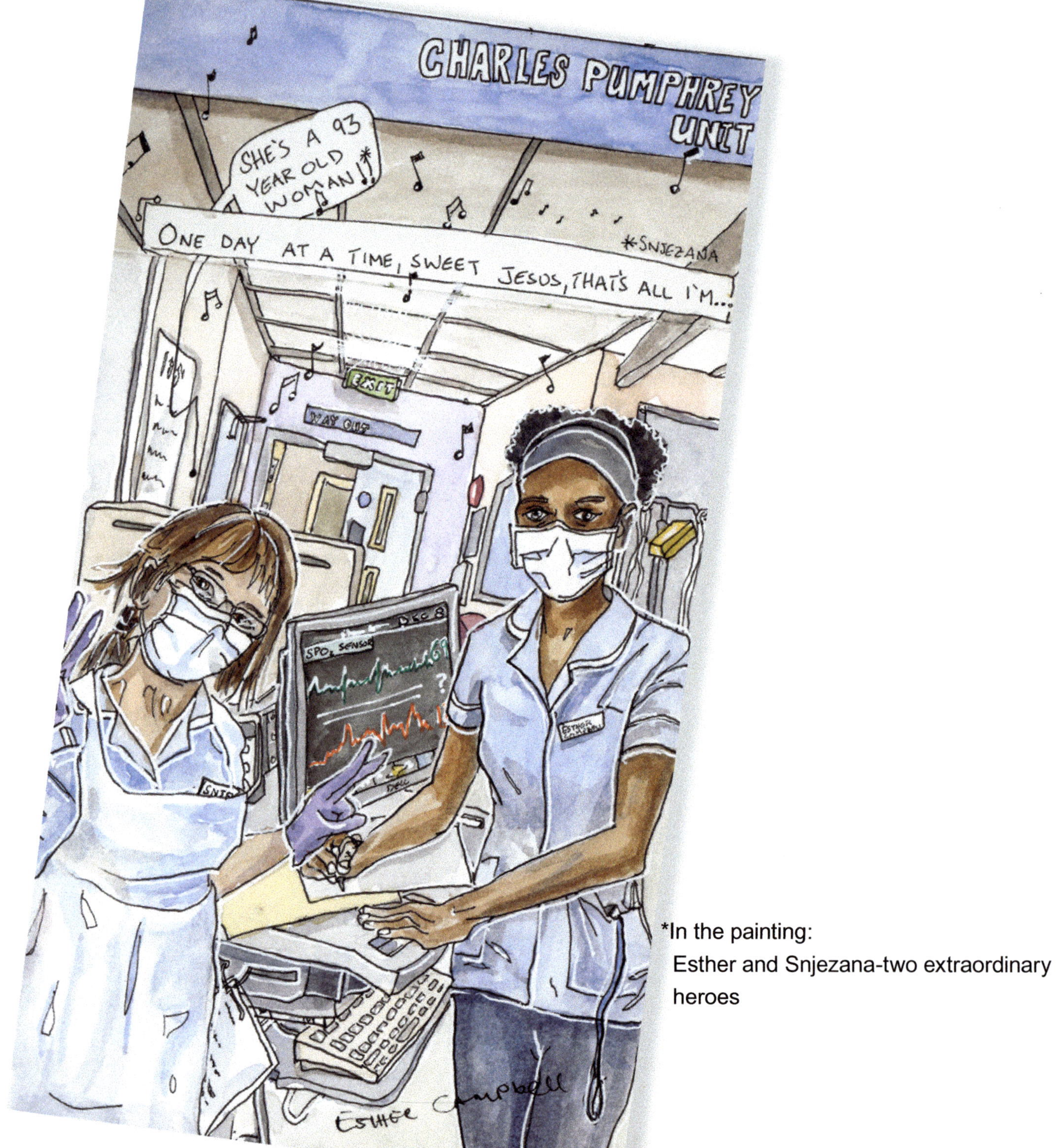

*In the painting:
Esther and Snjezana-two extraordinary heroes

I'M GOING TO DIE

"I'M GOING TO DIE."

"I'm dying. Help me. Please."

When we talk about 'heroes', the only way to really understand the true meaning of the word is to experience grace at their hands. It feels unearned and yet, it comes, seemingly without effort. It was the middle of the night, when the most profound things seem to happen. I was awoken quite suddenly and whisked unexpectedly to a new room – 'E-bay'. (I chortled to myself in a semiconscious state, wondering if I had won some kind of auction.) The nurse who was pushing my bed explained that I was being moved to a ward where everybody had tested negative for COVID. She had clearly had one hell of a shift; she was slightly dishevelled, hair a frizzy mess, and yet, she was still smiling. You could see it behind the mask, in the way her eyes kindly narrowed. She neatly wheeled me into my new parking spot and, with hopeful reassurance, she said, "It should be a little quieter here for you."

Then, she disappeared.

As my eyes slowly closed to reunite me with my night's slumber, I heard a faint groaning. At first it was low and unrecognisable, but then it grew into discernible words. "Help me, I am going to die." It was Manuel, a 90-something man, grey in colour, with a weak voice. "I'm dying, help me!" His cries grew, and a nurse glided over to his bedside. After examining his monitor and lightly stroking his shoulder, she reassured him that it would be alright.

The cries continued, throughout the night! Sometimes it was full-blown wailing, other times it was sorrowful crying, and with others, it was repetitive moaning. It would stop briefly as he fell into a shallow sleep but would restart again after a short kip. It would morph into new iterations, "I need food! Foood!" or "Help, I need help!" I was CROSS. And tired. And frustrated. I wanted to bellow out, "Stop talking, you ungrateful wimp!" But I didn't. And throughout, the nurses continued to go over to his bedside and reassure him. Despite all the other needs to which they had to attend, they just continued to support Manuel (and all the rest of us). The nurses themselves had sore backs, their feet hurt, and they were exhausted. They did not have time to complete their endless reports. And yet, they served us, usually with a smile, regardless of circumstance. Each of their patients was treated with dignity and respect — true masked crusaders!

DEATH VS TIME

OBSERVING human beings in an isolated microcosm is a worthwhile experience. During my time in hospital, I was confined to a bed, and so was forced/given the opportunity to observe the comings and the goings, the nuances and the grand gestures of people. At times, I was surprised by human nature and its ability to transform the lives of those within its sphere. Take 'The Turk', for example. Rotund yet sturdy in form, he was a seasoned man, one who had seen the world. Granted, he struggled with an impressive catalogue of ailments – bowel cancer, indigestion, constipation, emphysema and general grumpiness (my diagnosis). However, he, too, was a player. My initial impression was that he was a polite, generous man. Asking for help with warmth and responding with a well-oiled, apparently heartfelt, Middle Eastern, "Thank you so much." However, his true nature slowly oozed out. His constant buzzing of the call-bell echoed throughout the ward as his list of requests grew exponentially. Inevitably, the staff were not able to grant all his pleas, and so his requests turned into demands. The demands became increasingly more patronising, dismissing the nurses with flicks of the wrist and gnarled words. The atmosphere shifted dramatically; a sense of unease wrapped its calloused fingers around the ward. At one point, in his stewing anger, he turned to one of the nurses, and in a horrible low growl seethed, "I don't want to talk you anymore. Go away. I'm finished!"

Not only was everyone in the vicinity disgusted but their spirits were withering, including 'The Turk' himself, who was being sucked down a spiral of self-pity. That was death.
That was what causes heart attacks.

And so, I quickly determined to be a student of 'life'. To search for a quality that restored and healed. Fortunately, it did not take long to find it. It was in one small act: TAKING TIME. Taking time to listen to another person. Taking time to empathetically dialogue with another human being. Taking time to encourage a fellow patient. Taking time. Intentional, meaningful time.

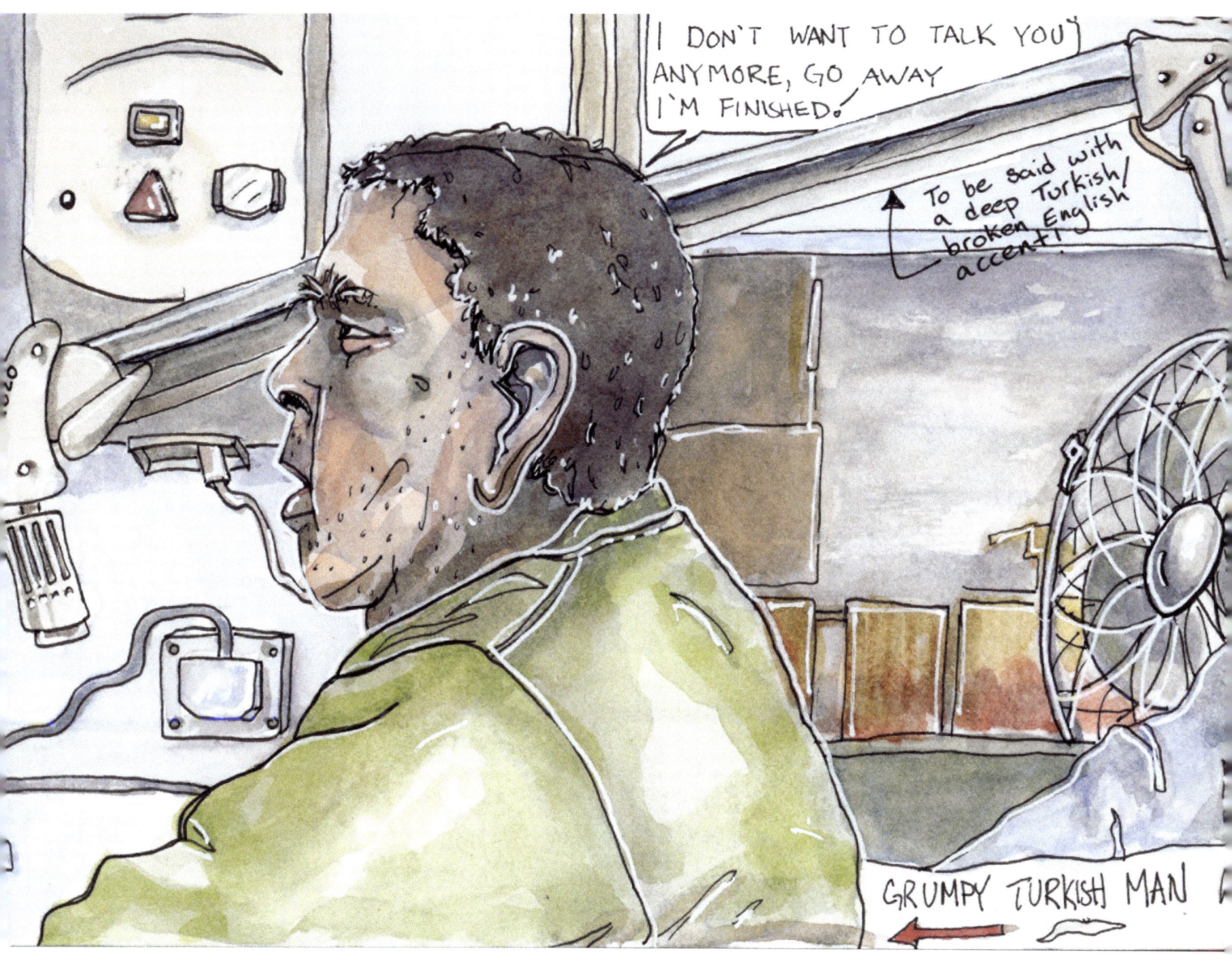

I DON'T WANT TO TALK YOU ANYMORE, GO AWAY I'M FINISHED.
To be said with a deep Turkish/ broken English accent!
GRUMPY TURKISH MAN

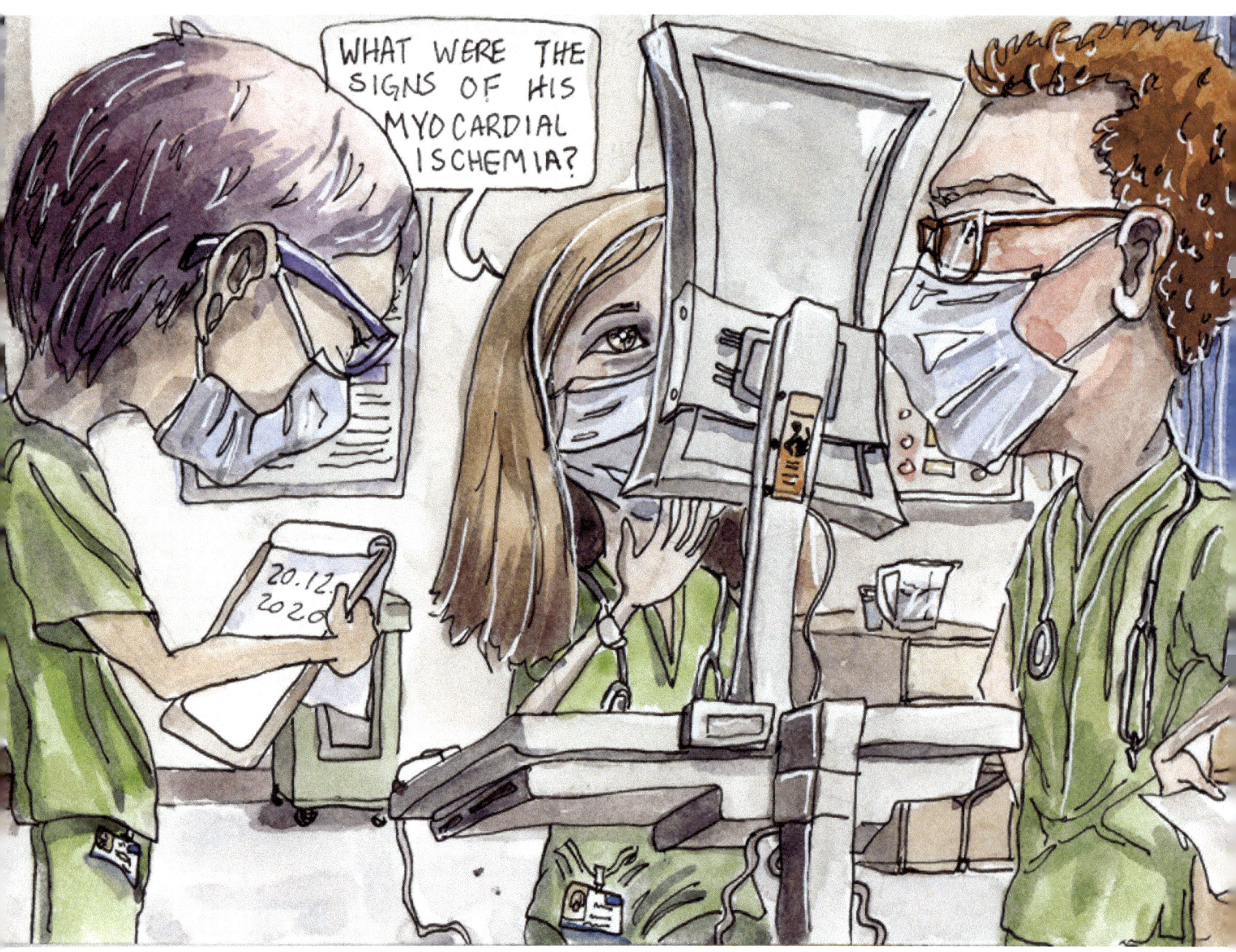

WHAT WERE THE SIGNS OF HIS MYOCARDIAL ISCHEMIA?
20.12. 2020

'DEEP' IN DISCUSSION

THEY WOULD ARRIVE, sweeping in like an Imperial Admiral flanked by her army of loyal Storm Troopers. The armada would float from bed to bed, discussing a few pointed questions, then regroup and, speaking in hushed tones, would discuss the fate of each hopeful patient. I watched, coyly eavesdropping as a lead consultant would grill the juniors and interns. You could see the exhilaration in the learners' eyes, desperate to draw the correct conclusion (and to impress). At times, a divine bolt of inspiration seemed to illuminate the situation, while at others, there was a process of narrowing and refining.

It was clear that this is how modern doctors are made.

But watching this has caused me to wonder, is it because of this intense peacock dance that modern medicine has come so far?

Many times, while in hospital I found myself in awe as science had once again miraculously found a solution to treating an otherwise impossible problem. The use of a perfectly dosed drug to stabilise a patient in seizure, the ability to observe the circulatory system live with echo technology, the innervation and repair of the heart, accessed by sending a microscopic tube through the tiny radial artery in the wrist. Quite frankly, it is awe-inspiring (and I am extraordinarily grateful). But it brings me to question if all of this, with its majesty, the 'miracle' of modern medicine, is here because people over the ages have met together in deep challenging discussions, pushing the limits of science, or is there something higher, more magnificent at work, guiding us and healing us together, as a human race?

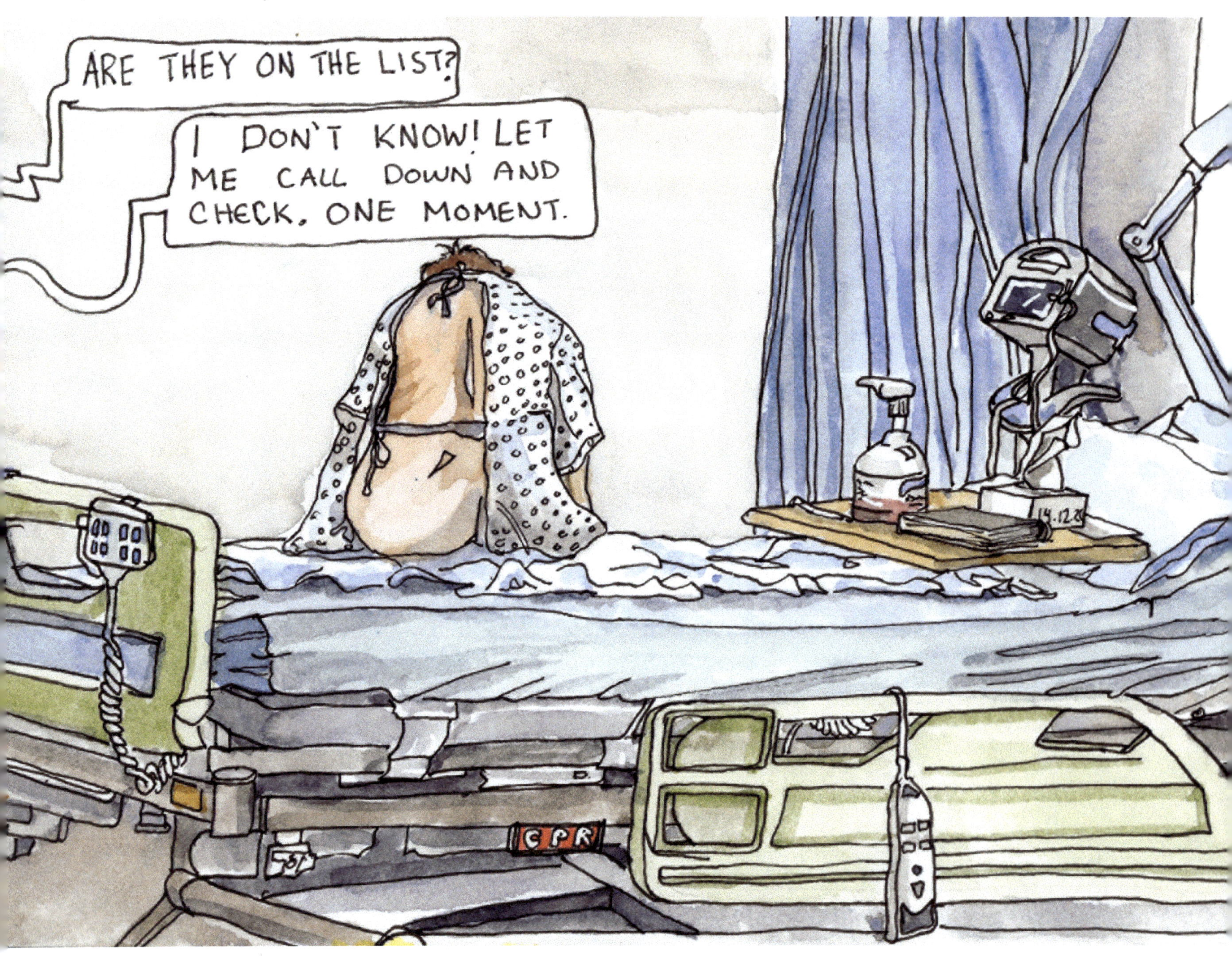

ARE THEY ON THE LIST?
I DON'T KNOW! LET ME CALL DOWN AND CHECK, ONE MOMENT.
CPR

THE LIST

TO BE OR NOT TO BE (on the list), that is the question. In hospital, each day brings a renewed sense of anticipation. In these places of healing, things are busy, they operate on a highest need, highest served basis. So, unless you are about to bleed out or are otherwise in imminent danger of death, your number necessarily slides down the priority list. Very logical. Add COVID to the equation and things get trickier. Extra lead times needed and medical staff off due to quarantine issues, and 'the list' gets longer. I was a significant enough concern that I needed to remain in hospital in order to get crucial tests (and possibly a procedure) done, so I was definitely on the list! Each day, a delightful nurse or doctor would look at their important clipboard or high-tech monitor and dangle the very real possibility of my number coming up. It was hanging there like a juicy carrot in front of an ambitious pony. It always felt in reach, and yet it was, in all reality, a good distance off. It became a daily topic of conversation. We would lust after the possibility. 'The list' became a magical entity. In my mind I could clearly imagine the day my name emerged victoriously. An angelic chorus of doctors would sweep into the ward and herald my name from a gilded parchment for all to hear!

Some days we lost hope.

But then, usually without any prior notice or ceremony, a doctor would arrive, and with a flourish, would pull the blue hospital curtains closed and tell you that it was your time for a test. When my moment came, it truly felt like a gift from the gods! I felt triumphant! I could not fight the smile that eagerly pulled at the corners of my mouth. But then, as porters expertly wheeled me out of the ward, my comrades enviously looking on, there was another feeling ... an odd feeling, the sudden realisation that not only was it my turn, and with it all the associated risks, but I was no longer on 'the list'. It had been the source of whimsical comfort for days, but now it felt like my membership had been revoked, tearing away the security blanket of the known.

It was now just me and the reality of 'the test'.

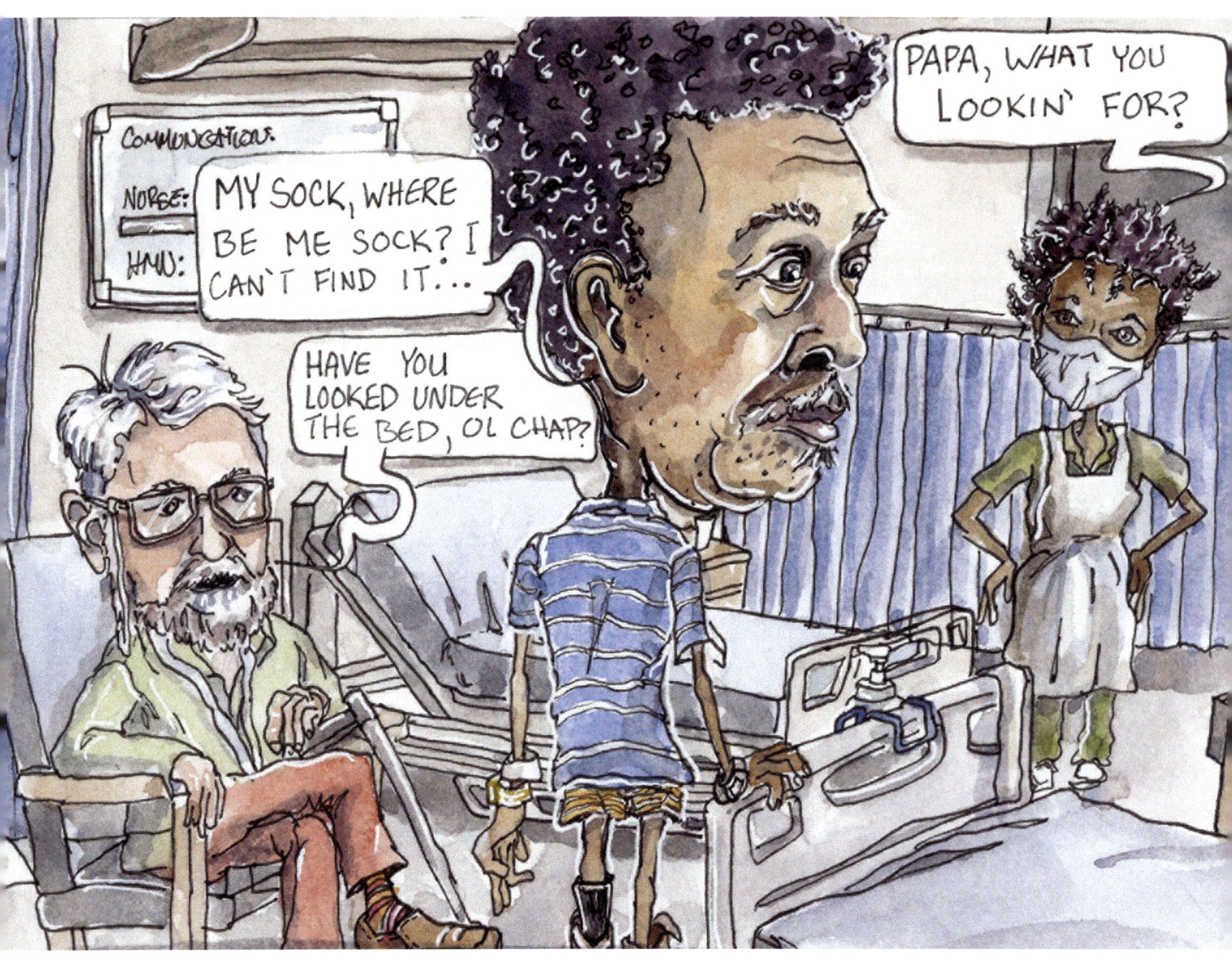

COMMUNICATIONS:
NURSE:
HMU:
MY SOCK, WHERE BE ME SOCK? I CAN`T FIND IT...
HAVE YOU LOOKED UNDER THE BED, OL CHAP?
PAPA, WHAT YOU LOOKIN' FOR?

MAROONED

I REMEMBER watching the film, Cast Away with Tom Hanks. I remember imagining myself marooned on a desert island, without human contact, succumbing to fear, loneliness and dissolving hope. I remember watching as Hanks's character, Chuck, hungered for relationship, to the point where he developed a bizarre, and somewhat comical, relationship with Wilson, an unsuspecting volleyball.

I remember watching a harrowing interview with an Iraq war veteran struggling to acclimatise back into civilian life, even with the support of his family, after having lived shoulder-to-shoulder with his fellow soldiers in the brutalness of war.

I remember finding myself in hospital. Suddenly plunged into an unknown world with a broken heart. I did not know the extent of my affliction; I did not know how long I would be there nor the residual impact on my life. I was, for all intents and purposes, marooned. Gradually, I found myself searching for and attaching to the people all around me. That was strange as many of them were not my usual cup of tea. Beside me was Bernard, affectionately known as 'Papa'. He came into hospital after being found naked, wandering the streets of Streatham. He spent day and night on repeat, looking for his lost black sock. While across from me, sat, the pontificating libertarian, who, by his own account, "A jolly dedicated civil servant in the House of Lords." The nurses came and went, each seemingly from a different corner of the globe. And yet, despite all these differences, they were community, and they provided safety in the shared experience of the hospital. On day five, when I found myself laying in the 'holding pen', alone, before my 'procedure', I felt fear tangibly creeping in. In the hollow bowels of the hospital, I laid in an empty cold room, a fluorescent bulb aimlessly flickering above my head.

Loneliness.

It was in that moment that I craved the security of home – my wife, my beautiful wife – and children. And, in that moment, I even missed my ward mates, 'Papa' and 'the Libertarian'. Humans were definitely not designed to do life alone on an island.

THE FEELING OF DEATH

PART 1- THE ICE SERPENT

MY HEART was already beating strongly when my stretcher was thrust through a sturdy set of doors into the cavernous theatre. As my eyes adjusted to the sudden onslaught of florescent light, I scanned the room. It was sparsely furnished. The cold palette of the catheterisation laboratory, ageing machines and clinically clad occupants reminded me of a Soviet-era military lair.

I was wheeled to the edge of a narrow sturdy table in the centre of the room and asked to shuffle my body across onto the platform. Once in place, there was the sound of snapping latex gloves, whispers, and the adjustments to machines. Then, we waited. I glanced at a wall of darkened glass; I could just make out the silhouettes of figures sitting behind blinking monitors. The delay only served to escalate the tension. After a dramatic interlude, the cardiologist entered through a side door flanked by an eager apprentice.

Clearly experienced, he made a few adjustments to the machines, checked the monitors and lowered his stool. Delicately grabbing hold of my right wrist, he introduced himself in a deep, considered voice, "Hello… (searching his notes) Mr Schmidt, my name is Doctor Kahn. I will be performing the procedure on you today." It was at this point that he rattled off an abridged version of the consent form that I had already (not really) read. He was well spoken, and he clearly knew his business, but the clinical approach combined with the unsavoury list of risks tangibly raised my anxiety. He finished with the kicker, "and there is a very small chance of death." I squirmed. In an effort to mask my fear, I awkwardly quipped, "I suppose I needn't worry; you've probably knocked out one or two of these procedures before, eh?!" He glanced over his Tom Ford glasses, clearly not amused.

The gist of the procedure is to find out if the blood vessels that innervate the heart are blocked or damaged. To accomplish this, they use a miraculous combination of electromagnetic radiation and microscopic cameras to assess the damage.

Doctor Kahn pulled a plastic-coated screen across the table and began his work. The local anaesthetic injected into my arm took effect in seconds. I was now a reluctant observer in this long anticipated surgical intervention.

A scalpel appeared, glistening in the theatre lights, before coming to bear on my wrist. Blood burst from its vessel like a pent-up geyser, spraying the transparent shield with a single crimson line*. My left fist clenched as the gravity of the situation became clear. Quelling the bleed with some gauze, the doctor then inserted a cannula, allowing access to the radial artery.

This manoeuvre enabled the next two stages, neither of which were particularly enjoyable. The first step was to inject an iodine contrast. The apprentice warned me that it was normal to feel a cold sensation moving through my body. I prepared myself. Then, gradually, I felt it slither up my lifeless arm like an icy serpent malevolently creeping towards my heart. My fist clenched again, and I closed my eyes. I could feel the fluid enter the chambers of my heart. My body was rigid with fear. "Just breathe, Mr Schmidt," a gentle voice reassured me as the radiologist manipulated his robotic camera towards my chest. "Take a deep breath. Now hold it … and relax. Again … " After a canon of these images were taken, I was left to rest as the team analysed the photos. It did not take long before they spotted the problem. Nestled snuggly in the left anterior descending artery was a small, curious patch of plaque occluding the vessel. They swivelled the screen to show me. There, in black and white, was a singular gnarled, unwanted lump blocking the flow.

My heart sank.

*Plastic waste has always been a bugbear for me. I often feel it is quite unnecessary, and
for the sake of our planet, we should minimise its use where possible. However,
on this occasion, the disposable plastic film was clearly fit for purpose!

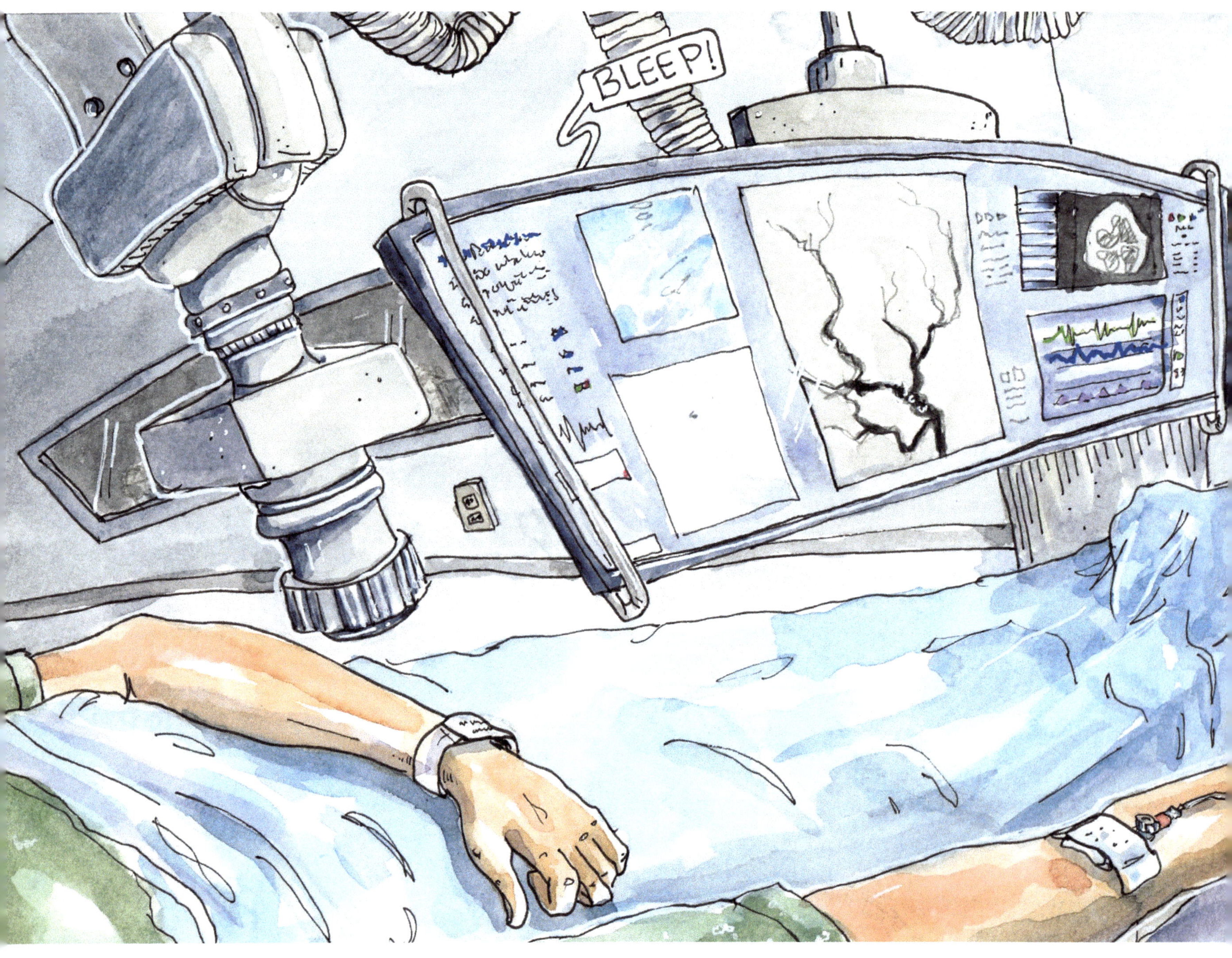

BLEEP!

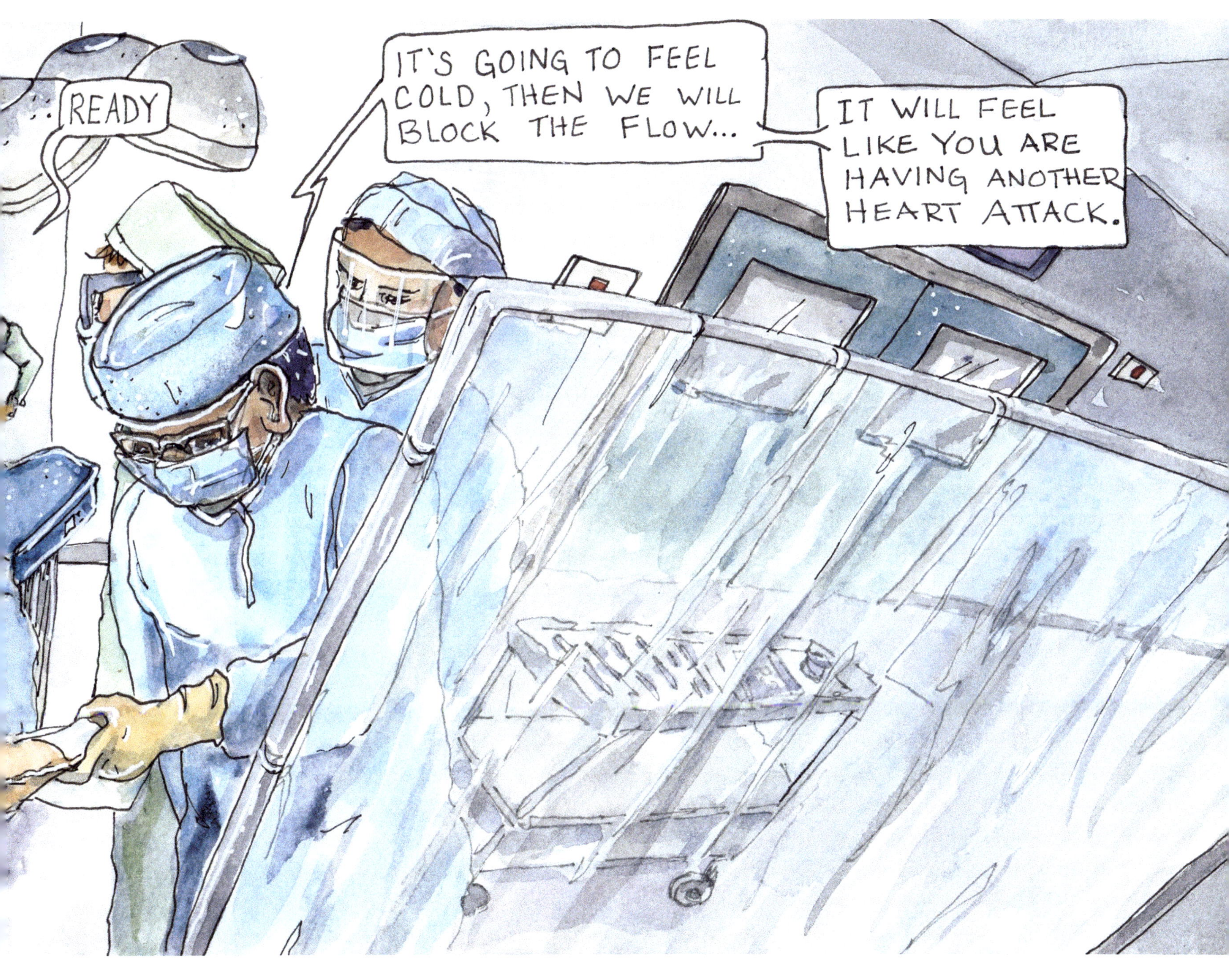
...READY
IT'S GOING TO FEEL COLD, THEN WE WILL BLOCK THE FLOW...
IT WILL FEEL LIKE YOU ARE HAVING ANOTHER HEART ATTACK.

THE FEELING OF DEATH

PART 2- ANOTHER HEART ATTACK

AS CASUALLY AS A WAITER might offer coffee after a meal, the doctor flatly asked, "Would you like to have a stent fitted?" Previously, in the ward, the doctors had spoken about the possibility of stents and by-pass surgeries, but I had quickly dismissed those ideas as fiction. After all, I was a 'fairly' heathy chap and certainly too young for such interventions.

"Do you want a stent?" He repeated. I lay precariously balanced on my little table under the glaring lights, left to make a spontaneous decision. I definitely did not have enough information. So, I blundered through a series of questions, blurting them out as they came to me; "What would my quality of life be like with a stent? What is a stent? How is it inserted? Is it lifelong? Would it corrode?" Time was not on my side, and I had to decide. I asked one final question, "What if I don't have it done now?" The doctor responded by saying I could very well end up in the same position in the near future. The very thought of enduring this process again was too overwhelming. So, on what felt like a whim, I agreed. And they set off to work.

The act of guiding a tightly coiled mesh tube through a network of blood vessels to be inflated via a microscopic, catheterised camera is, quite simply, a miracle – but not without cost! My nerves faltered and were no match for the steely concentration of the surgeon. My body braced as I focused on a tiny silver bolt holding together the monitor above my head. Doctor Kahn guided the probe towards my heart and proceeded to explain what would happen next, "When the stent arrives at the blockage, I will inflate a balloon inside the implant which will expand the mesh but will also block the artery. In that moment it will feel like you are having a heart attack again, but it will only last for about 10–20 seconds then you will return to normal." Fear instantaneously grabbed hold.

"I'm going to inflate the balloon now." Doctor Kahn warned.

I began to breathe quickly as I prepared for the induced attack. It came on slowly, the pain creeping across my chest like a thousand cords cinching in unison. The memories of days earlier were now vividly flashing through my mind. Panic! Involuntary shaking took hold. Is this what death is like? Is this how I die? The medical team reached out to calm me. Sweat, like dew, appeared on my forehead. My toes curled and my eyes squeezed shut. Then, at the peak of the tension, came release. As quickly as it had arrived, calm swept over my body as the adrenaline dissipated.

What had started as a good idea, resulted in another brush with death and ultimately a life-altering procedure. These encounters with mortality are deeply felt and often painful, but I feel they should not be wasted, rather they should help us to live our lives better.

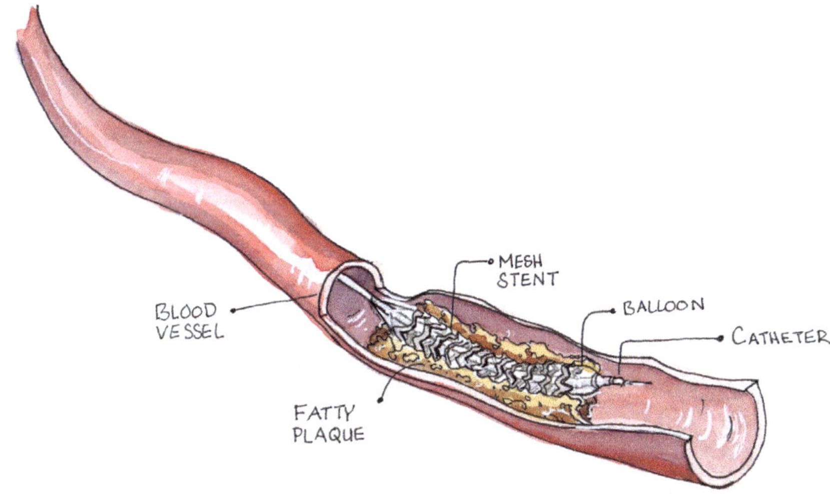

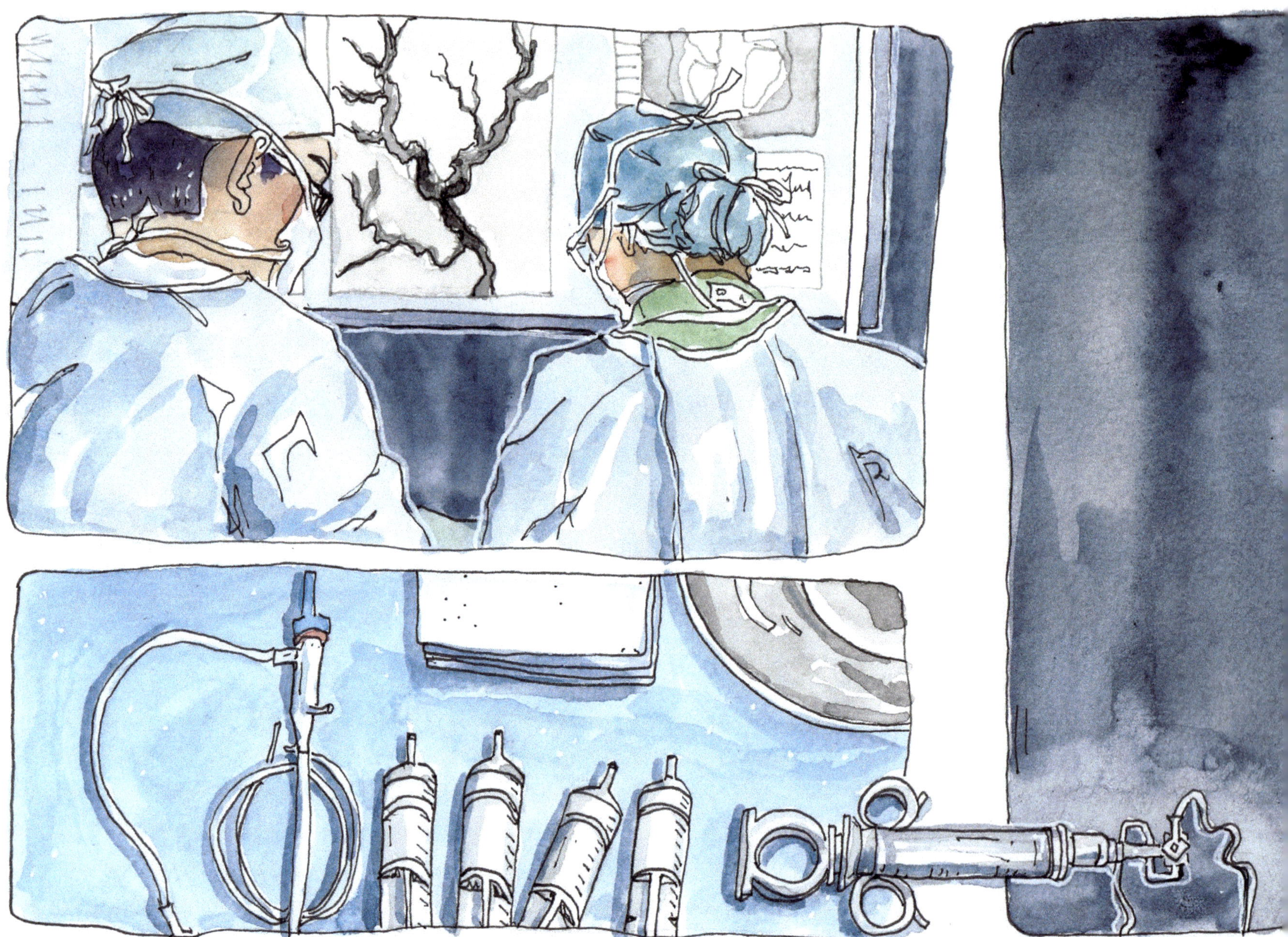

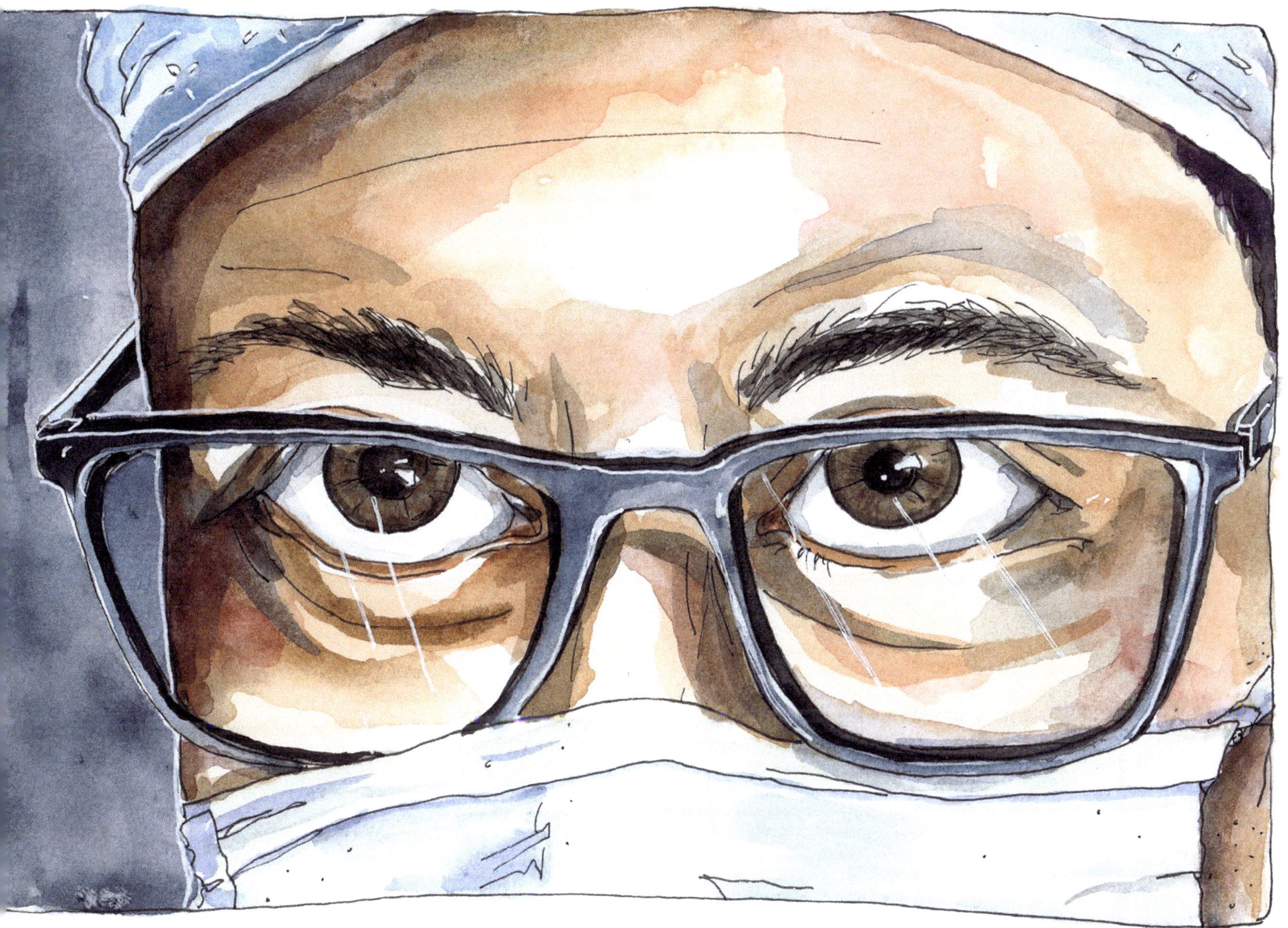

DISPLACED INTO THE WILD

OVER THE DURATION of my stay in hospital, I saw many people come and go. Observing this daily migration had become a familiar part of my routine. It was fascinating to see patients make their dramatic change from standard-issue hospital gowns into the clothes they had arrived in; it was a sort of time capsule hailing back to the moment of their crisis. Many times, their personal attire added another layer of colour and understanding to their personalities. 'The Libertarian', for example, transformed from his green uniform into a debonaire Harris Tweed jacket, punctuated with a mustard yellow bow tie and magnificent red trousers. As he shuffled out of the ward, he tipped his trilby and wished us all "a jolly fine stay."

The day finally came for our little band of brothers to end the adventure. Although David was the first to get his stents fitted, the doctors felt that they needed a little more time to observe him. So, it was Mark who led the way. With his implants in place, he made his final wardrobe change and was almost unrecognisable in his street gear. We all said goodbye, making informal plans to reunite. But despite our smiles, it all seemed rather quick and unceremonious.

Then came my turn. Despite days of waiting in what now felt like home, I was surprised to find that it was only hours after my procedure that I would be released.

I changed into my jeans and button-down shirt, slid on my cardigan and laced up my shoes. As I sat awkwardly perched on the end of my mechanical bed waiting for my discharge notes and medication, I had the distinct feeling of being displaced. My hospital routines had become so familiar and safe, and now I was to be released back into the wild.

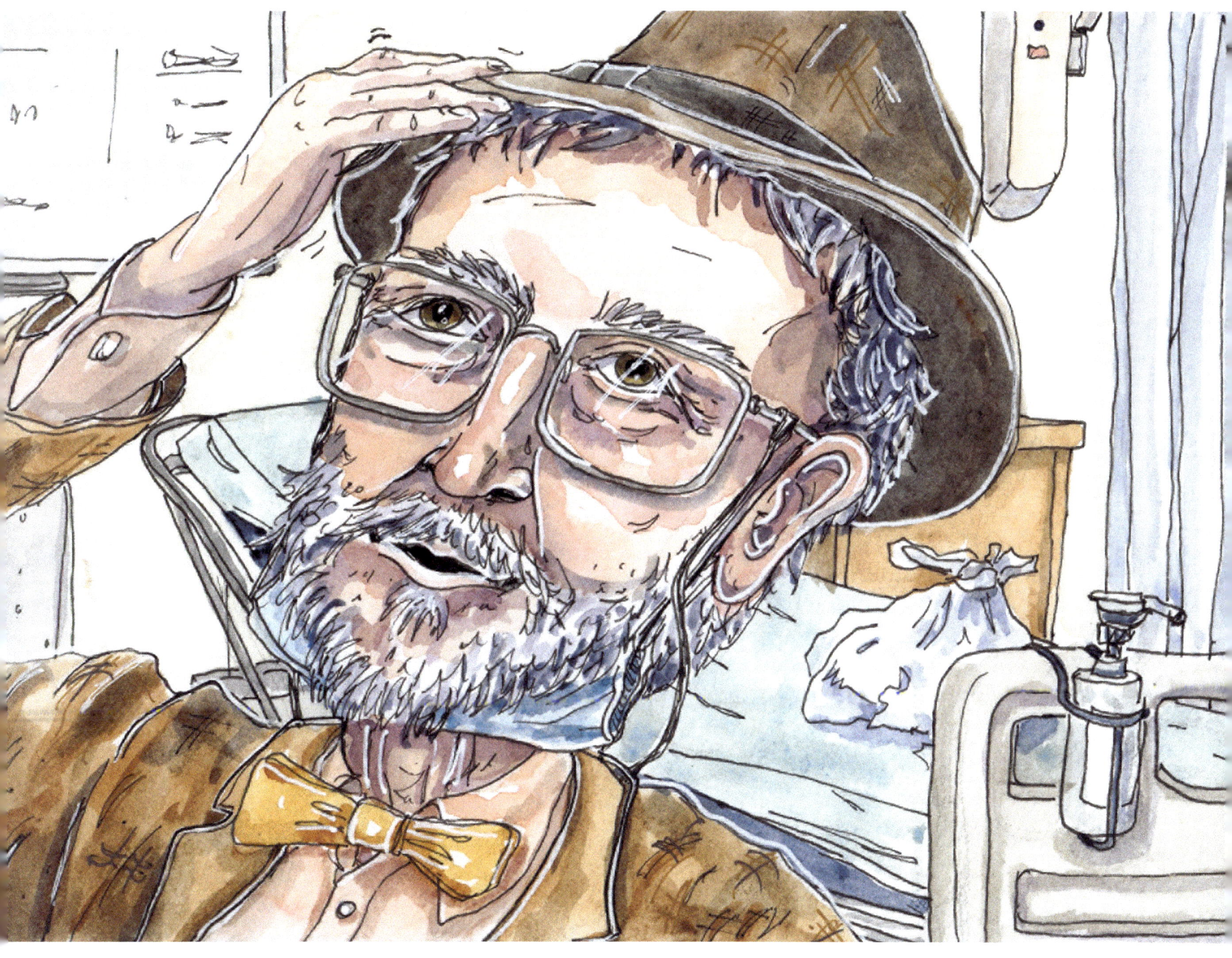

After a very rushed consultation with the matron, I bravely walked out of the unit with my little rucksack and an armful of drugs. I felt somewhat jilted. I had not even had the opportunity to properly say goodbye to the nursing staff.

It was much colder outside the ward, and I wished I had worn another jumper. As I made my way to the elevator, I was keenly aware that the hospital was a frantic bustle of activity. I felt invisible and lonely, and ordinary. I was no longer the high priority patient of hours earlier, and, with no visible signs that I had experienced any sort of trauma, I was just another guy. The elevator doors slid open, and a porter glided out pushing an elderly woman in a wheelchair. I smiled hopefully, but they were unmoved. I stepped into the lift, pressed a button and descended to the ground floor. Then, quietly making my way through the warren of corridors and clutching my medication, I wondered if I would be alright.

At the peak of my melancholy, I looked up and spotted my wife who was waiting outside the main doors (she could not come in due to the COVID pandemic). I could see her face from a distance, her compassionate smile beaming at me. My heart fluttered within my chest. As I drew nearer, I paused and turned to take one last look at the hospital foyer. There were various staff attending to others' needs (no longer mine). In that moment, I saw that for these workers, unlike for me, there was no time to rest or reflect. My feelings of self-pity continued to erode, being replaced with a rising tide of gratitude; how blessed was I to have had an opportunity that made saying goodbye so hard! I shivered again before a warm embrace ... and a new beginning.

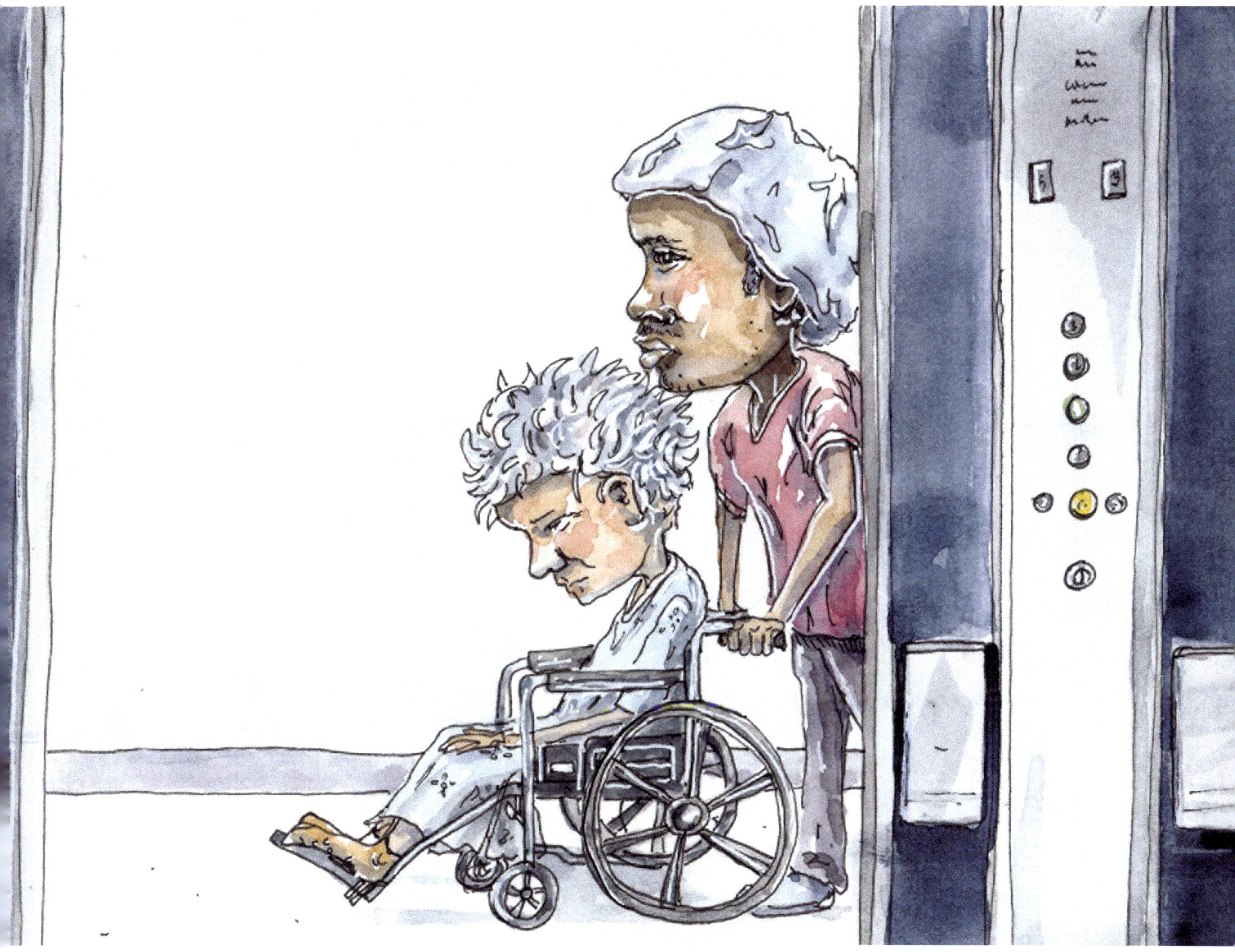

Recovery

THE ANTITHESIS

MY HEART ATTACK really was a spot of bother in the masterplan of life; it was the kind of blight that brings all forward thinking to a screeching, definitive halt. Although it came at the climax of the academic term, in reality, it was probably due more to the culmination of a life of fast living. It's an approach, some deep narcissistic belief that I have the superhuman ability to 'squeeze a quart into a pint pot'. I remember, years ago, my mum remarking, "This pace you live is unhealthy. You can't possibly sustain it!" I responded by inflating my chest and exhaling a finely crafted "guffaw" – just enough to acknowledge her comment but insignificant enough to let her know that she was clearly mistaken.

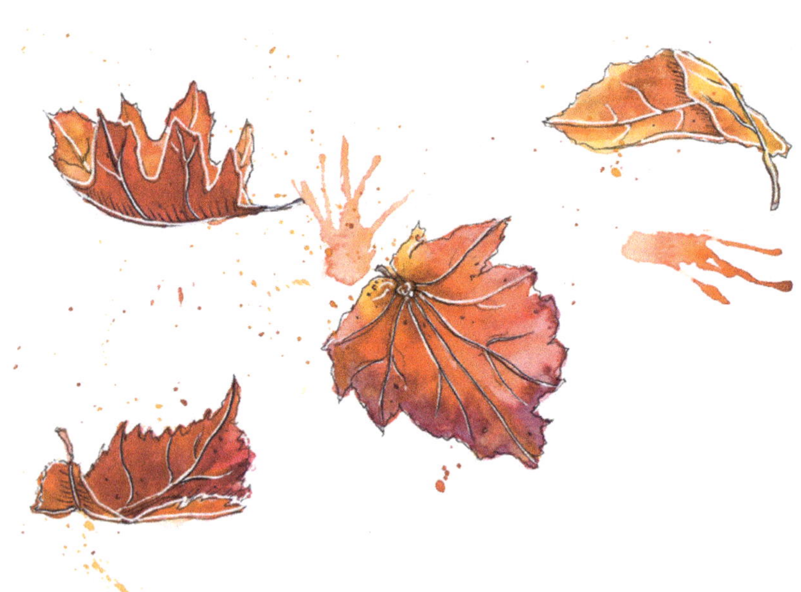

Now, at 46, I sit in the humbled company of the delusional, forced to swallow a bitter pill of defeat. *

However, it isn't all bad. When forced to slow down and reflect, I found a growing clarity. Increasingly, I am able to spot the beauty in the simple things in life. For instance, sitting out in front of my house, legs crossed, the romantic vista of the Surrey Hills stretching out endlessly ahead of me, I am gently reminded of the carnal words of the seclusive Scandinavian, Markus Torgeby, "Your heart is worth listening to. Each heartbeat supplies your body and mind with the (necessary) oxygen they need." As I slowly take a sip of my finely brewed coffee, contemplating life, my new journey starts by listening to that subtle, profound guiding beacon tenderly beating inside my chest.

*To be precise, at the time of writing, a concoction of eight unpronounceable tablets.

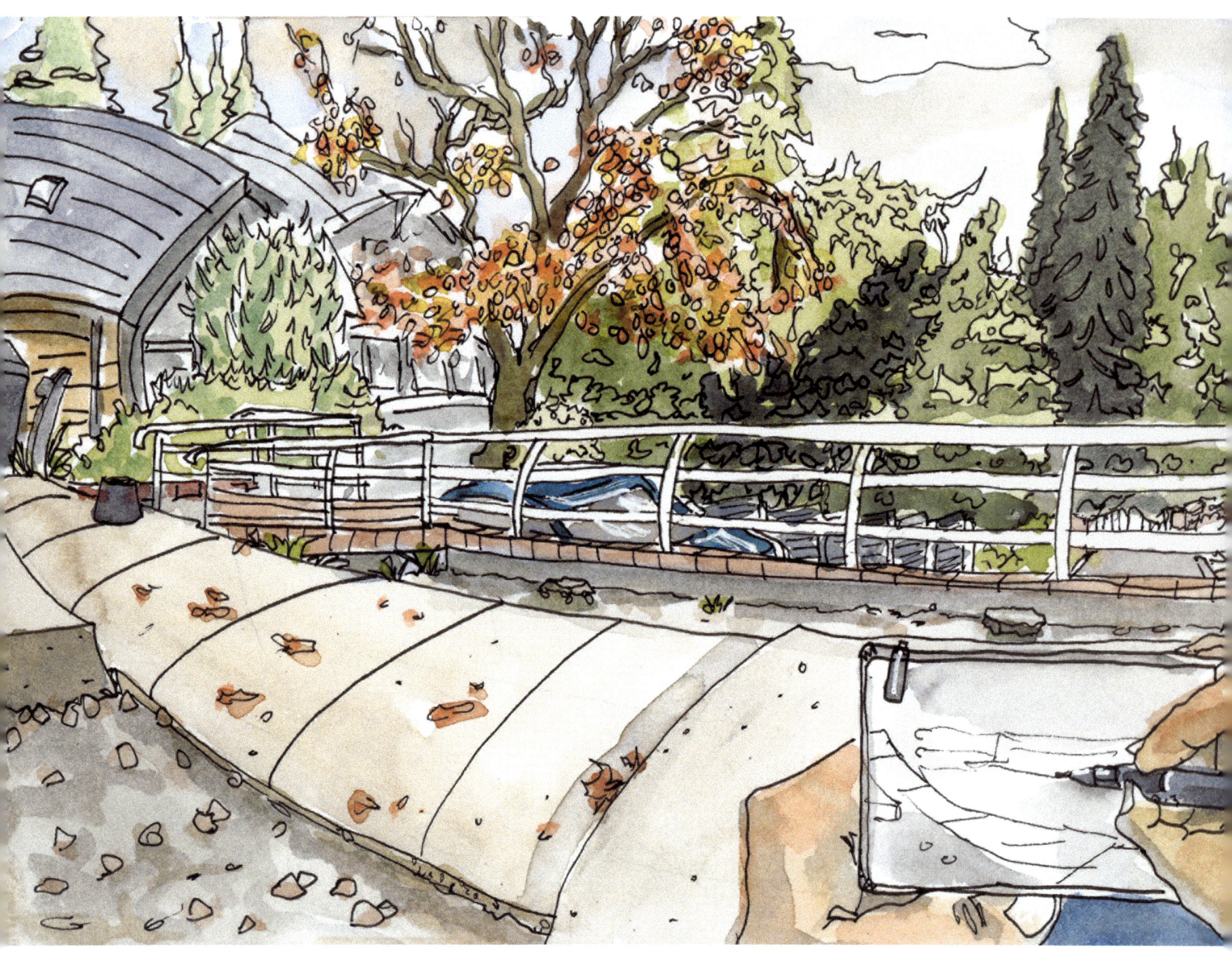

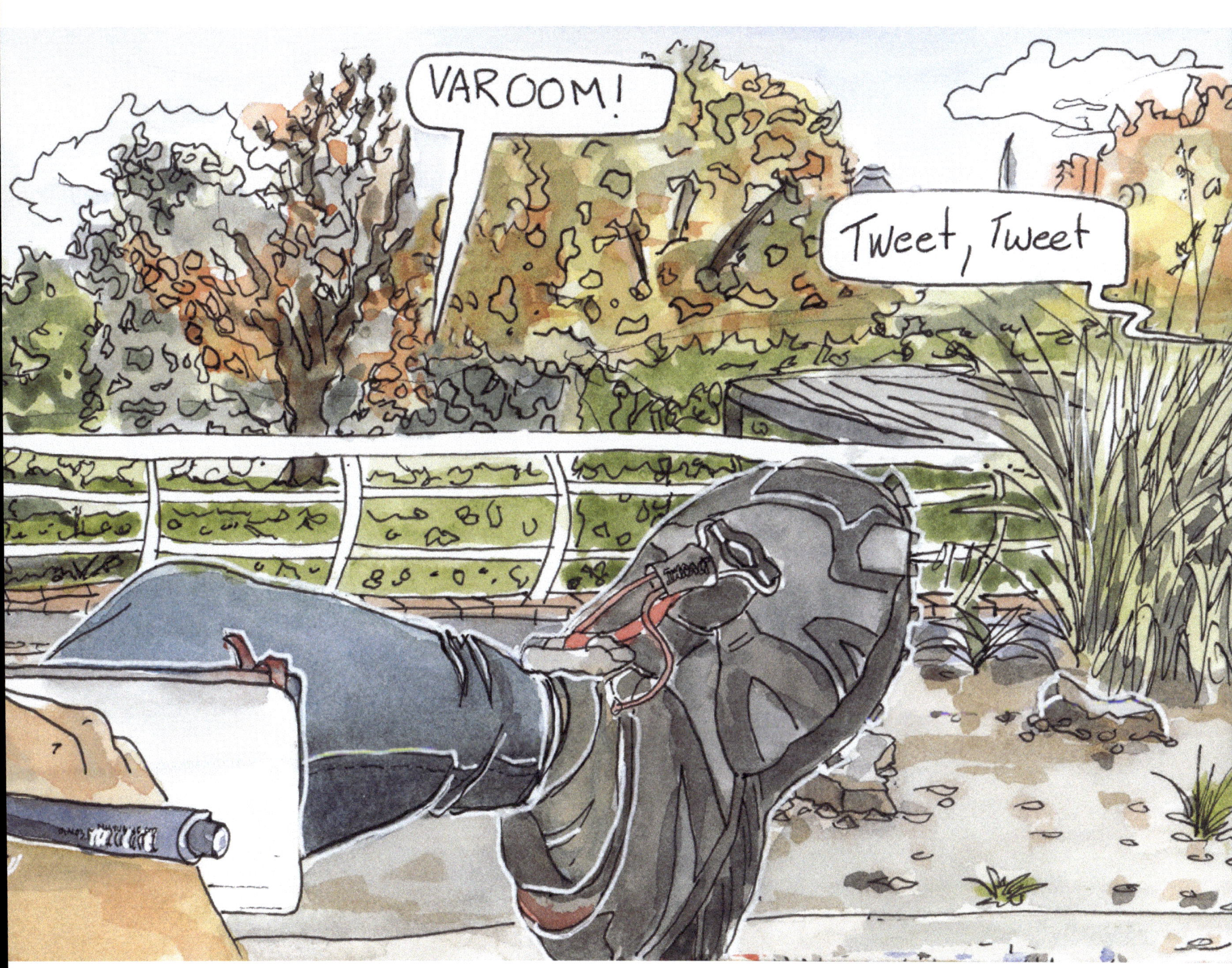

VAROOM!
Tweet, Tweet

THE SOURCE OF LIFE

BEING IN RECOVERY mode has been a revelation on various levels. For starters, sleep has gone a long way towards restoration; with eight plus hours each night, my dreams are no longer fraught with difficult decisions and battling ferocious beasts. Instead, they have been thrilling and optimistic, transformed into epic James Bond-esque adventures. In my waking hours I can think more coherently; I effortlessly enjoy time with my family, have longer conversations in which I am 'present' and have found joy in things long abandoned. Take reading for example, recently (and embarrassingly) an arch nemesis of mine. It has been my tepid goal to read one book a year (because 'it is good for me'). I usually attempt this on holiday and with great reluctance. However, in one week I managed to read one whole book, voraciously. And started a second!

I am also observing more, and putting those observations to page, allowing my paintbrush and pen to tell the story. I get lost in that world – observing architecture, weathered by time, and the people, bustling about, lost in the lists of their day. There, in that place, I can feel my heart soaring, like the kestrels that float effortlessly on the rising air currents above my house. That artistic act is the fuel for poets and the stuff of proverbs. So, this is now my mission, to guard my heart – physically and metaphorically – as I re-enter modern life, post heart attack.

"Guard your heart above all else, for it is the source of life."
-King Solomon

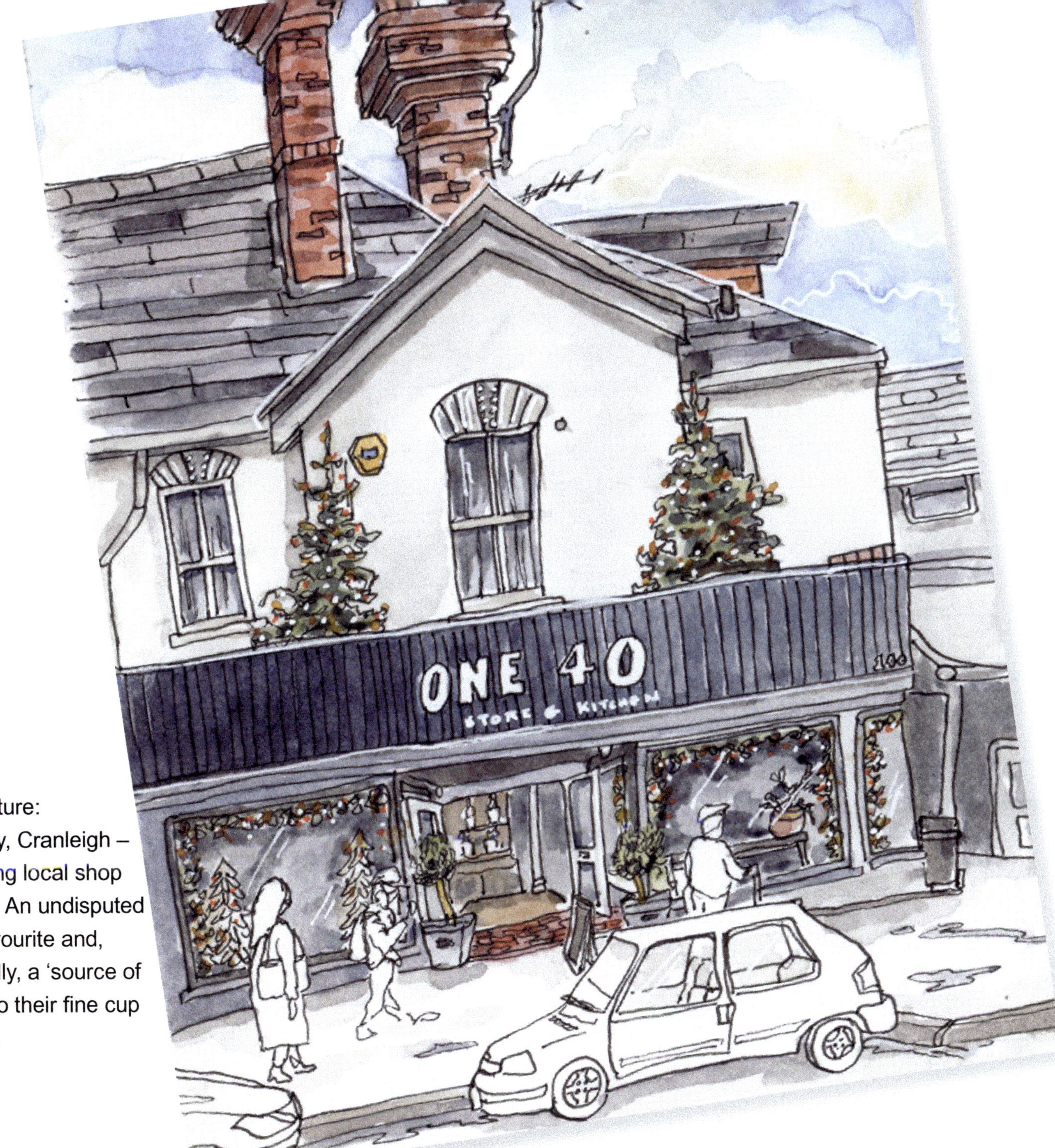

In the picture:
One Forty, Cranleigh –
a charming local shop
and cafe. An undisputed
family favourite and,
incidentally, a 'source of
life' due to their fine cup
of coffee.

UNDER AN OPEN SKY

IN MY all-things-are-possible teenage youth, I would have this fairly regular conversation with my dad, regardless of the season. It would go something like this:

"Dad, looks like a great night to sleep outside. You in?"

"Are you nuts!? Why would I want to sleep outside when I have a perfectly good bed inside!"

Even before asking the question, I knew the answer would be a flat, "No," peppered with some off-hand comment that would insinuate that I had a screw loose. I loved those conversations. Roughly translated (in my mind) that meant, "I love you, my great adventuring son!", which I greatly accepted, and even though I couldn't really understand why he wouldn't want to sleep under the endless canopy of stars philosophising about the infinite universe beyond, I gladly took those opportunities to commune with nature.

I am now a middle-aged working man, immersed in the roaring race of life, childhood a distant memory – until recently. In the weeks following my heart attack, my wife gave me a marvellous book which reminded me that living close to nature does something deep in one's soul.

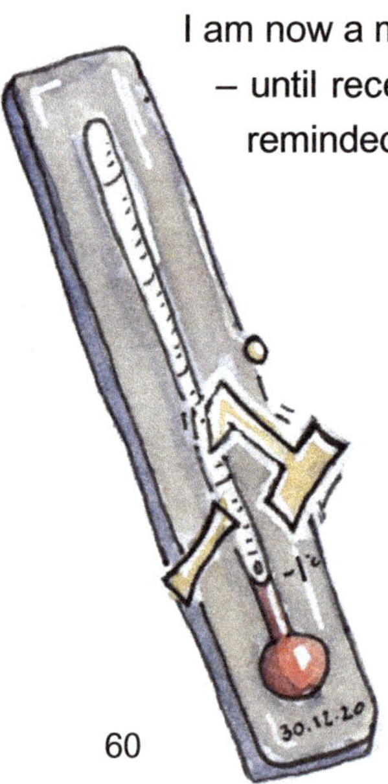

And so, on a whim of inspiration, I heralded an invitation to the family, "Tonight it will go down to freezing, a clear sky, it will be a great night to sleep outside. Who's in?" The response was, overall, positive; optimism perched on the plinth of adventure! And so that night, after explaining the science of sleeping bags and the magical healing powers of sleeping in the outdoors, the whole family joined me on the back deck. Within the ranks there was palpable excitement, and a dash of irrational fear. Would we sleep? Would Jeff's heart stop beating from the shrill cold? Would he die? Would we all die!? Frozen to death, five frozen corpses!? Regardless, the anticipation of the escapade pipped any looming fears. The prospect of deep, cosy warmth in the sleeping bags fending off the gnarly cold lured us in.

That evening, as the evening frost gently settled, the fragrant winter air filtering into our lungs, we all drifted off into a deep sleep…
…until 2 am, when a helicopter circled, reminding most of the party that they were sleeping outside in winter, and they had perfectly good beds inside.

They abandoned ship, leaving me to myself and the infinite sky above me.

Heaven.

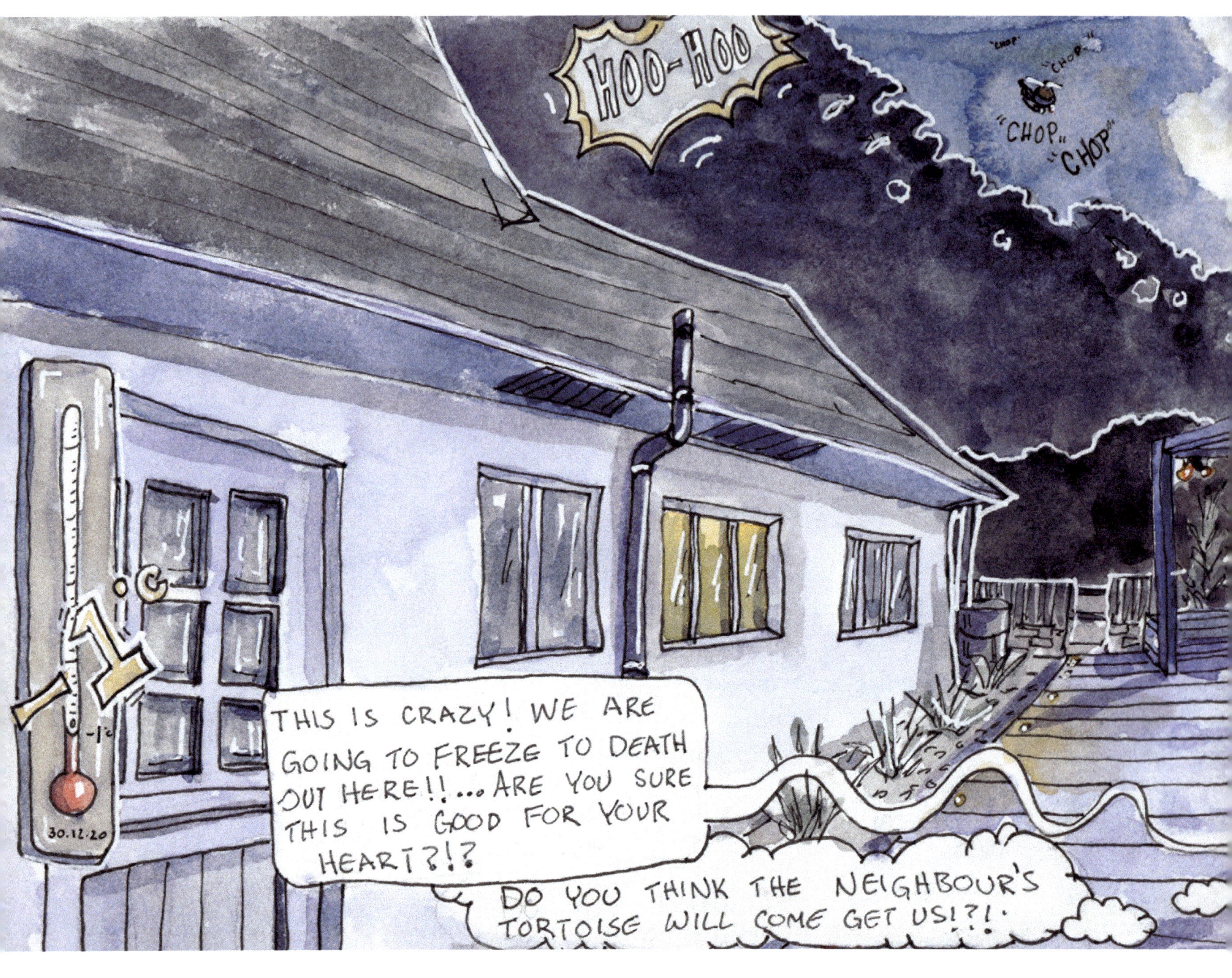

HOO-HOO
"CHOP"
"CHOP"
"CHOP"
"CHOP"
30.12.20
THIS IS CRAZY! WE ARE GOING TO FREEZE TO DEATH OUT HERE!!...ARE YOU SURE THIS IS GOOD FOR YOUR HEART?!?
DO YOU THINK THE NEIGHBOUR'S TORTOISE WILL COME GET US!?!

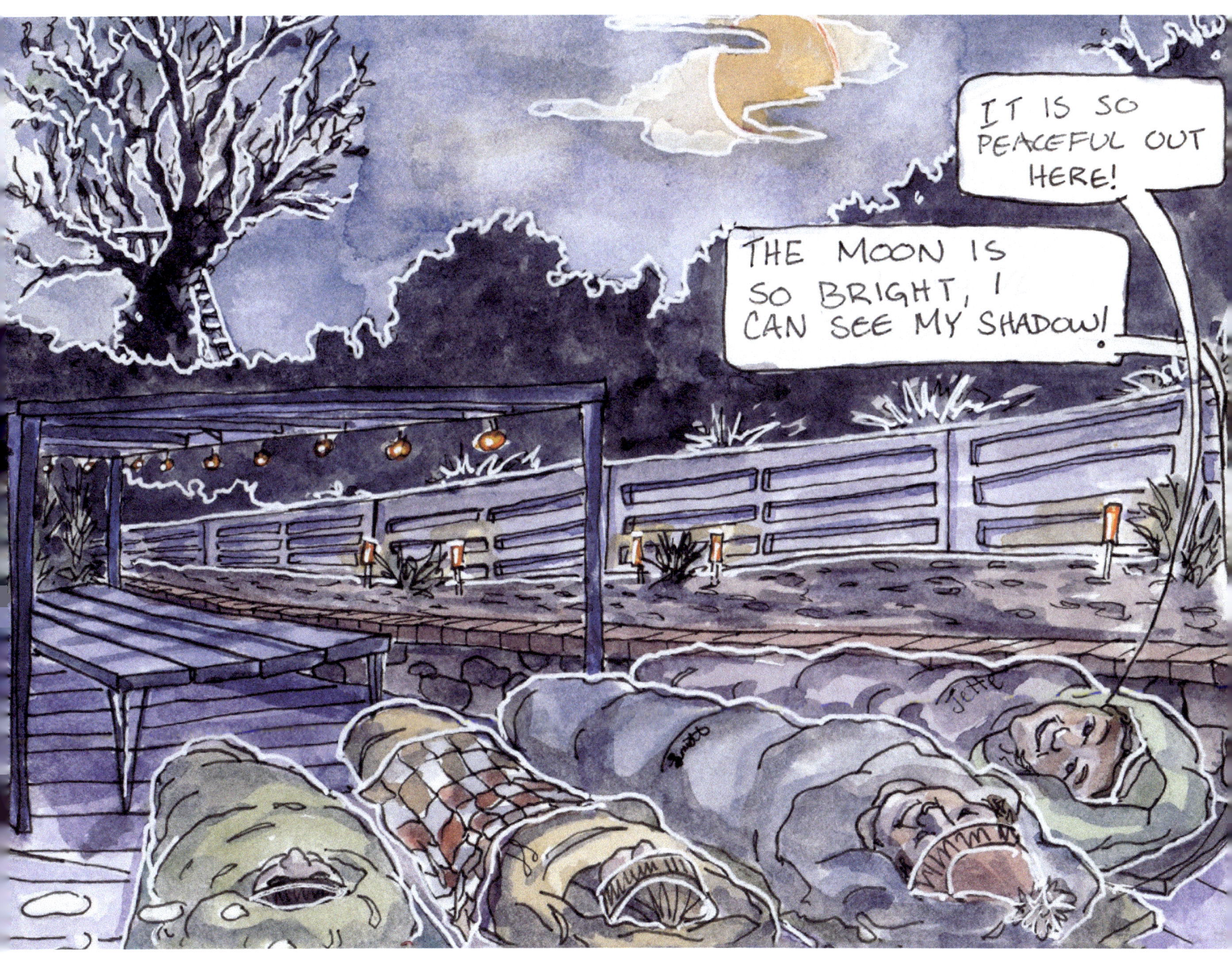

IT IS SO PEACEFUL OUT HERE!
THE MOON IS SO BRIGHT, I CAN SEE MY SHADOW!

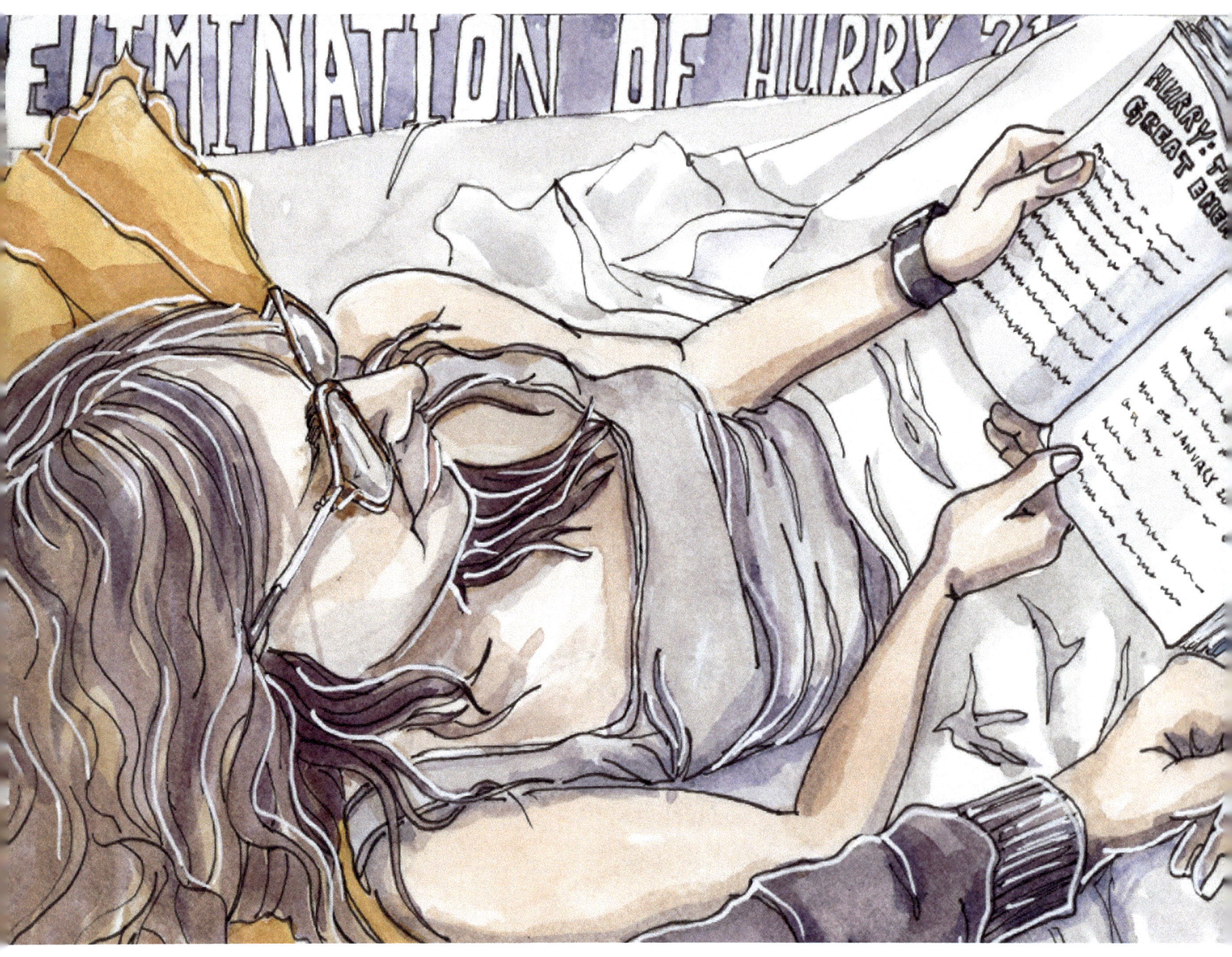
ELIMINATION OF HURRY
HURRY: THE
GREAT ENEMY
JANUARY

HURRY

"HOME NOW, LATE DINNER. Can't sleep; that dead-tired-but-wired feeling. Crack open a beer. On the couch, watching an obscure Kung Fu movie nobody's ever heard of, Chinese, with subtitles...I feel like a ghost. Half alive, half dead. More numb than anything else; flat, one dimensional. Emotionally I live with an undercurrent of a nonstop anxiety that rarely goes away, and a tinge of sadness, but mostly I just feel blaaah spiritually...empty. It's like my soul is hollow." *

How's that for an opening of a book? Depressing, definitely. But when it resonates, it's painful. I had been feeling this sense of uneasy imbalance for a while. My wife and I had even had conversations about it, highlighted by the various physical maladies I was experiencing. Restlessness. Gut issues. Back issues. Then, WHAM! A heart attack! I now know that I should not have been surprised, but I was. As time wears on, I have had people appear from various chapters of my life with their stories of burnout and trauma. Many similar to mine and thankfully some with tales of hope after the storm.

I had a heart-to-heart with a good friend, Chris, who interrupted me halfway through a chat and said, "Can I preach to you for a few minutes, brother?" (I should note that using the term, 'brother' softens the blow of any looming difficult conversations.) He went on to speak about stress, Jesus and yokes. It was good. Very good. It hit deep. I think he could sense the impact that his words were having on me and so he paused and asked for my address so that he could 'Amazon' me a book. I obliged.

When it arrived, I tossed the book in the pile of 'to reads' (quite a large pile) and sent a polite thank-you message. But over the next few days something kept pressing me, and when my wife saw it, well, it turns out that the title resonated with her too. So, we agreed to read the book, together. By together, I mean her reading aloud to me (heaven for both of us!). This is our new routine, a revelation! No Netflix. No phones. Just her and me, and a whole lot of wisdom. Something is happening deep within my soul.

*Excerpt from John Mark Comer's book, The Ruthless Elimination of Hurry.

A LIGHTNING-BOLT MOMENT

IT HIT ME as I sat snuggly nestled beneath the protective old stone fountain at the centre of town. I had cosied my back against an ancient pillar and was observing the world; people bustling to and fro under the gentle embrace of a vibrant night sky. It was there, and only fleeting, that I had one of those deep Weltanschauung (philosophical world view) moments, as though God himself had allowed a brief glimpse from his perspective.

I have heard it said that the two greatest gifts we can give our children are to be present and to love. Solid (and challenging) advice. But what else? I often think, beyond that, beyond meeting those deep indispensable needs, what is it that we need to pass on to our children? Ideas are never too far from the surface and if I stop to think about it, the list grows: give compliments freely and generously; joy is a choice; there is refreshment in the natural world; don't be embarrassed by your emotions; listen to the nudging of your soul; say "Thank you" to a compliment; drop the ego; say sorry (often). The list feels endless and overwhelming.

But in that moment, at the centre of our little village, it was as though time slowed down and I saw that 'what else?'. It was people. People enriching the space around them and connecting, each in their own way, to the world.

"You can only be you," I thought to myself.

And that was it, the lightning-bolt moment. It spoke to my heart. Pretty simple but liberating and life changing. I spend so much time thinking about what others have done, what others have achieved, and the meaningful contributions they have made, that I lose sight of who I am.

So, that night I lay down with my children and, as we reflected upon the day, I left them with this: "I want you to know that there is this awesome place where your passions, your gifts and your gumption collide. It's in that space where your soul thrives, others are blessed, and the world is a better place. Live that life well."

*In the picture: the peaceful village of Cranleigh under a vibrant night sky

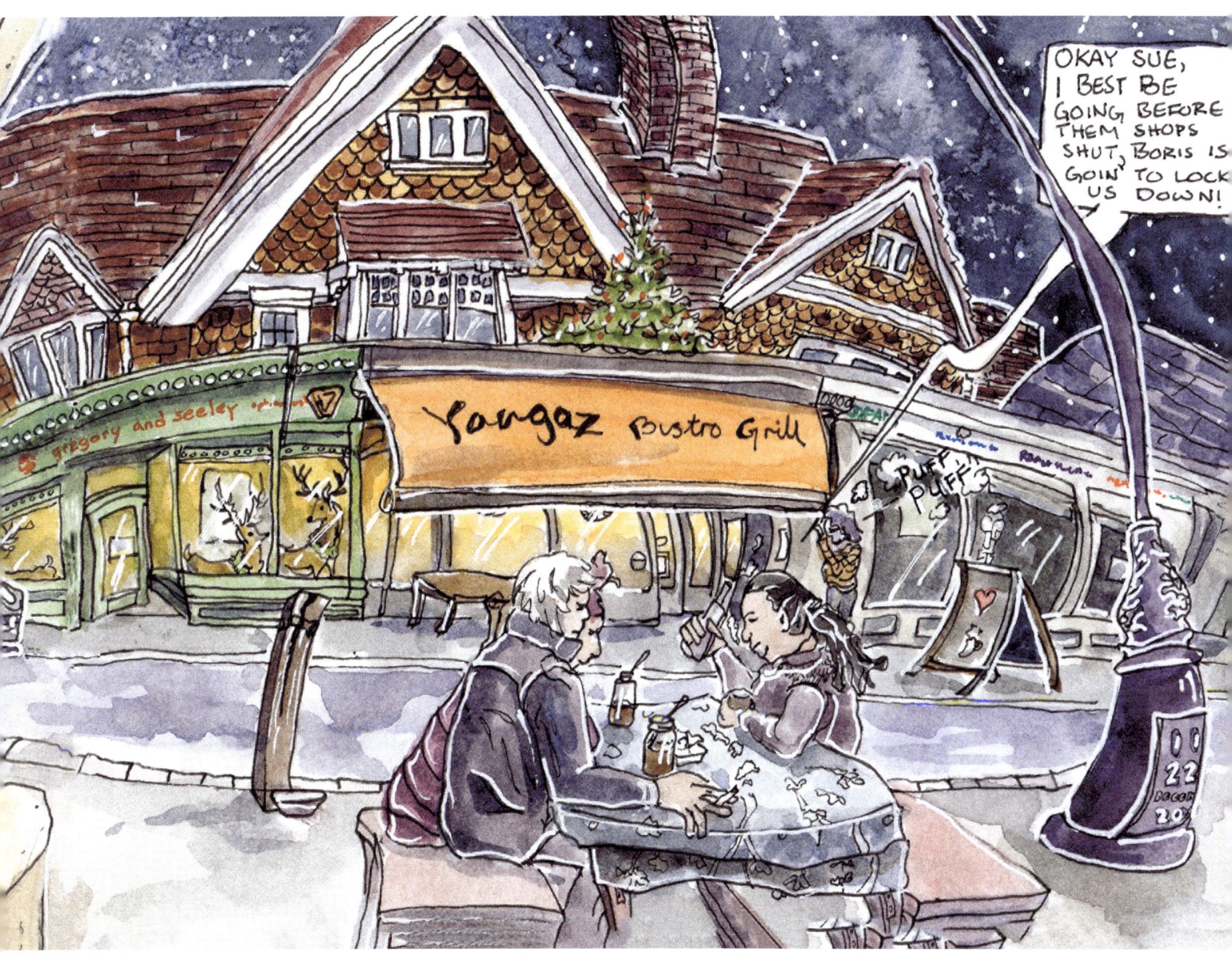

OKAY SUE, I BEST BE GOING BEFORE THEM SHOPS SHUT, BORIS IS GOIN' TO LOCK US DOWN!
gregory and seeley
rangaz Bustro Grill
PUFF PUFF
22 December 20

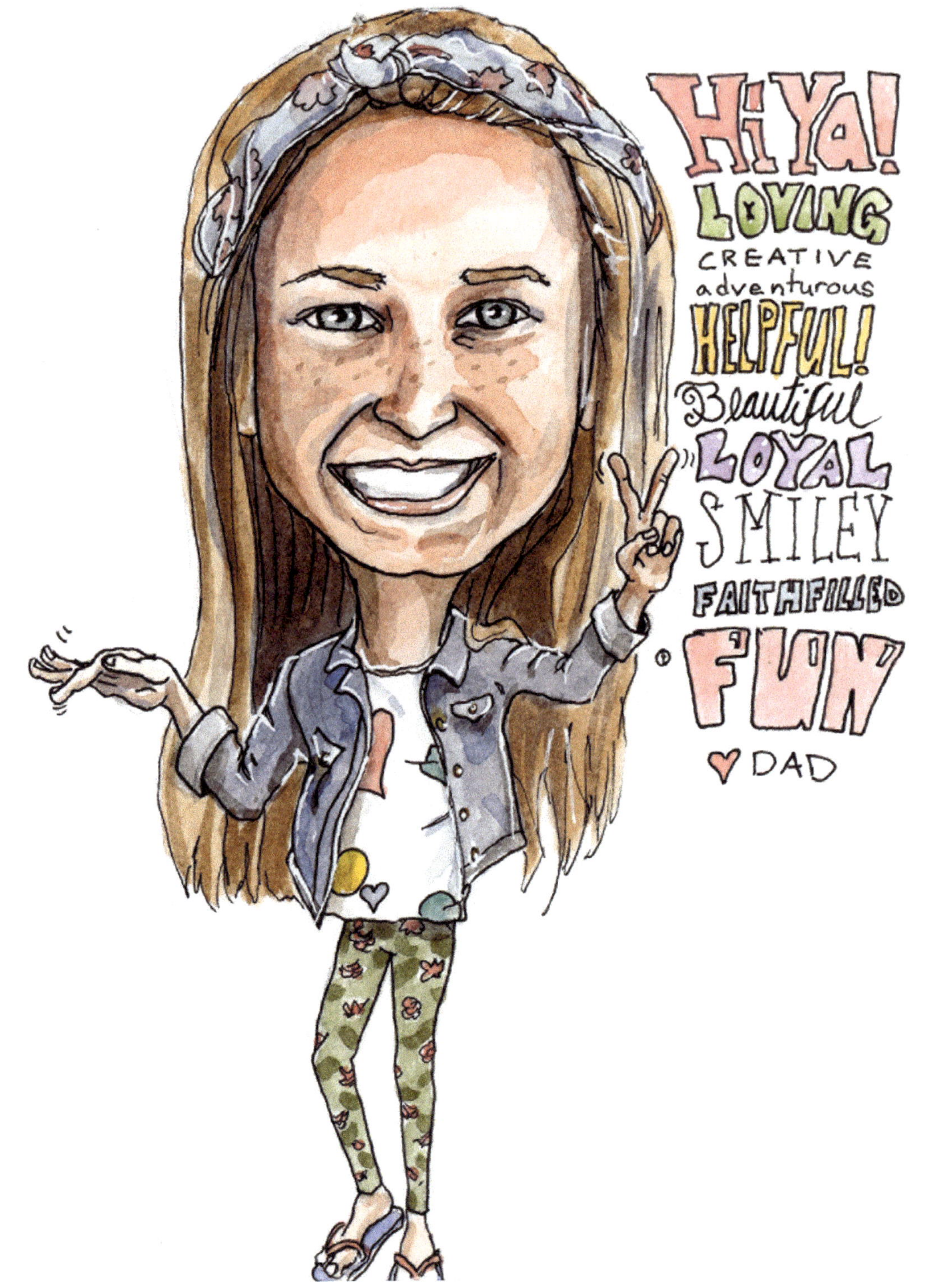

HiYa!
LOVING
CREATIVE
adventurous
HELPFUL!
Beautiful
LOYAL
SMILEY
FAITHFILLED
'FUN'
♥ DAD

SIMCHAH

THERE IS THIS BEAUTIFUL little word in Hebrew. It is not so much a suggestion as a commandment for how to live and, like so many other foreign words, it does not have an equal in the English language. Simchah refers to 'joy'. A deep sense of joy that infiltrates every chasm of life. And, quite crucially, it is shared. The belief is that when a person lives their life with joy, they are much more capable of serving others. This little nugget of a word was gifted to me by an unerringly wise friend early in my heart recovery. I was clearly wrestling with the elusive 'meaning of life' question and little did I know that discovering Simchah would be an important key to my journey.

One day in mid-December, my eldest daughter asked if I could paint her something, anything. She just wanted a painting from me. "No problem," I quipped, thinking I would just magic up a little flourish of inspired art. Certainly, she would be happy with anything I, her dad, made. But when I sat down to paint, I couldn't decide what to do. My brain filed through its dusty catalogue of ideas: cutsie gnomes, magical flower gardens, picturesque sunsets, reimagined pop-art, a puppy, or a horse. I felt like it should have been easier. I felt conflicted. A gift for her had to have meaning. She was my daughter, after all. She relies on me, counts on me to lead her, champion her and show her how to love. It had to say something significant. I wanted it to say, "You are joy!" So, in my angst, I did nothing.

Over the next few weeks my daughter continued to drop little hints, as she had not forgotten. Little comments that translated, "I am dying to have something special from you. I don't want to put any pressure on you, but I would really love a painting!"

Feeling quite desperate I went to the source of good ideas (and may I add, joy) – my wife. She simply said, "Why don't you paint a picture of her in your fun, comic style, with some words about how you feel about her?" Eureka! Yes, that was it. It flowed effortlessly.

And this is what I am learning. Find your Simchah, and it will flow effortlessly. Grow it and safeguard it so that you might serve the world around you well.

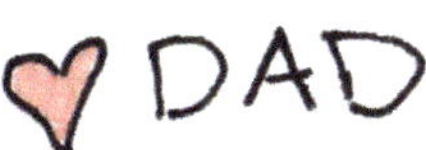

A CUP OF TEA

I UNDERSTAND, to some degree, the irresistible urge that prospectors and explorers must feel: the deep-rooted desire to give up everything and head into an unknown frontier in order to discover something new. I know it in the physical, in my adventures in the untamed wilderness, off the beaten path, pursuing the possibility that I could be treading on land previously unknown to human footfall. (I have always thought that is an extraordinary idea to be the first human to encounter a space.) There is great joy in venturing off the beaten path, getting lost, making discoveries, then finding your way back.

To my great surprise, my recent introspective adventures have yielded the same thrill.
As I sift through the (cobweb strewn) alleys of life, I have made many discoveries – some painful, others pleasantly effervescent. It is a funny thing trying to 'discover' who you truly are, who you have been designed to 'be'. It should not be that difficult, after all we live with ourselves 24/7. However, I have discovered that we all have blind spots. These unseen spaces, although obvious to those around us, are obstructed from our own view. Every so often the mist clears, and we may get a glimpse of these thorny suburbs. For instance, I have always embraced challenges and projects with flourish and gusto – 110% (apparently). An admirable quality, I think. However, when that drive becomes all-consuming and is then projected on and expected of those around you, it becomes unhealthy, even ugly. Looking back, I can see how some of my vain pursuits have unnecessarily ruffled feathers and deflated souls. Ouch.

I recently had a conversation with a good friend, I call her, 'the Reverend' for the simple reason that from her heart pours such goodness that I often think it is straight from heaven. She had popped by to drop off some heart medicine (homemade fudge!). I couldn't invite her in due to COVID, but, of course, she knew that and had come prepared. We talked from the doorstep. After a while she pulled up a stool and we continued to have a good ol' natter. The intended drop-off turned into a much longer than intended catch-up; she always has time for connection ... and tea.

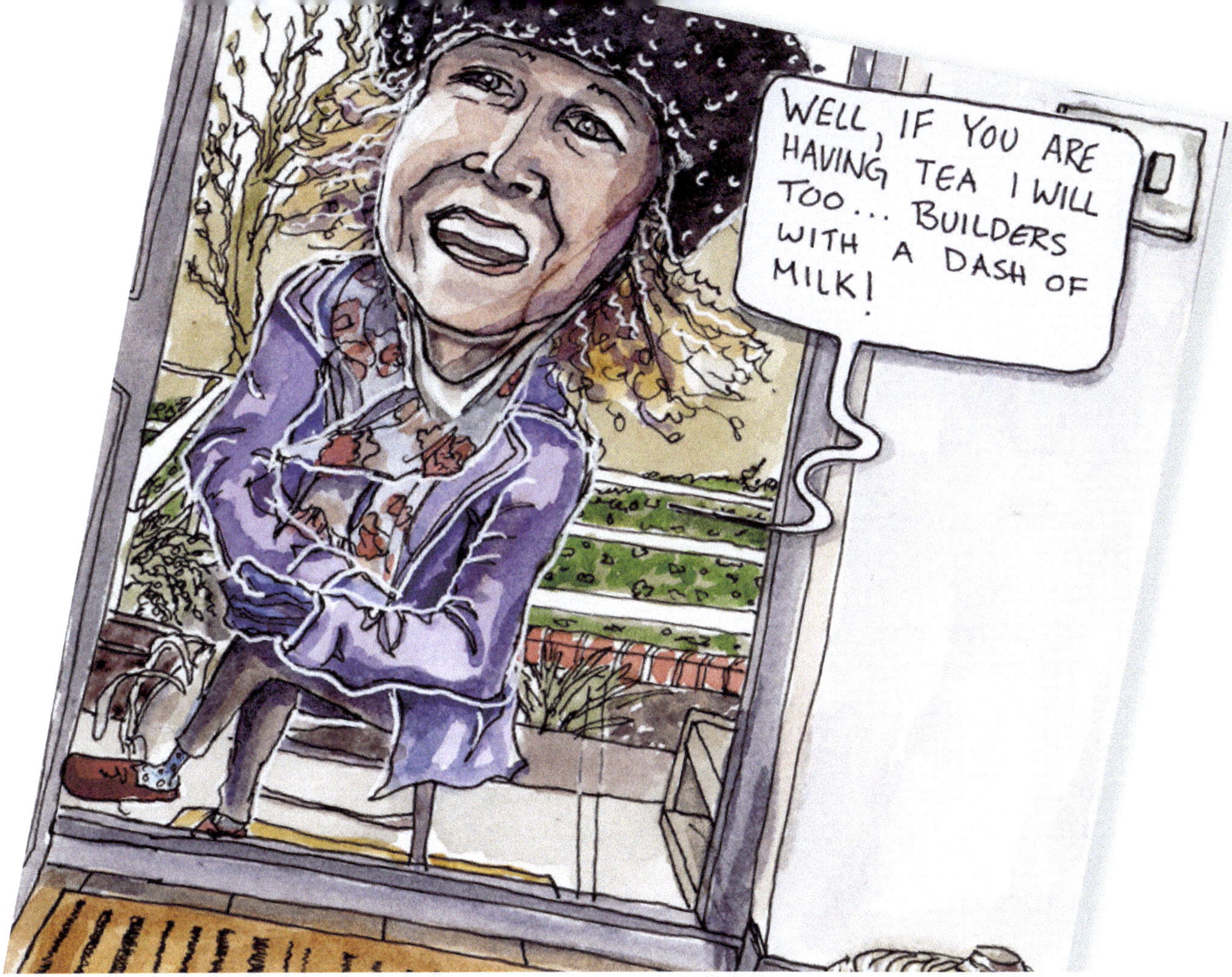

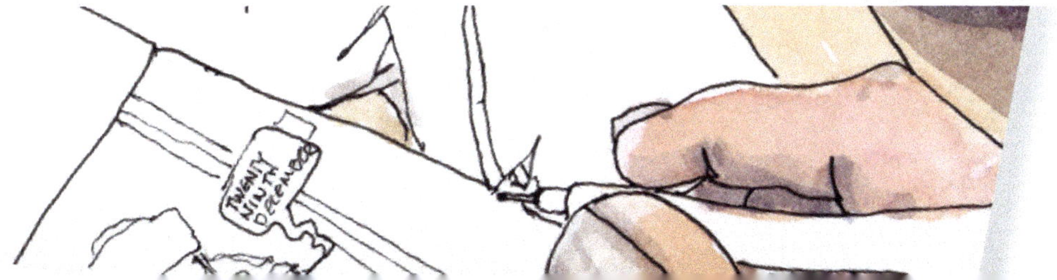

As an aside, tea, in my mind, has always been a pseudonym for 'leisurely conversation', which is something I haven't really ever had time for; it stands in the way of the next great breakthrough. But there it was, a long leisurely conversation, with tea. And, by Jove, the primitive discovery that leisurely connection with a friend is good; very good. Another blind spot revealed.

TIRING OF NATURE

IT WAS a Monday night and the darkness of winter had once again settled heavily over the hills. We were all in lockdown and the children were deep into a programme of online lessons. The shift back to routine was not easy and we yearned to return to the freedom of the holidays and joy-filled adventures. As the day drew to an end, I could sense the guileful power of the increased screen time, the artificial, flickering light slowly enveloping their consciousness, eyes glassy with an undertone of cabin fever taking hold. There was a clear need to remedy the impending infirmity.

I have been around long enough to know that the natural world has great power to restore balance, and so I quickly deferred to this time-tested tonic. It is widely accepted that, as humans, we have lived in close connection with nature for 99.9% of our existence on this planet. For millennia we have worked with the land, in seasonal rhythms that afforded us essential rest and refreshment. But with the invention of the lightbulb, life changed.

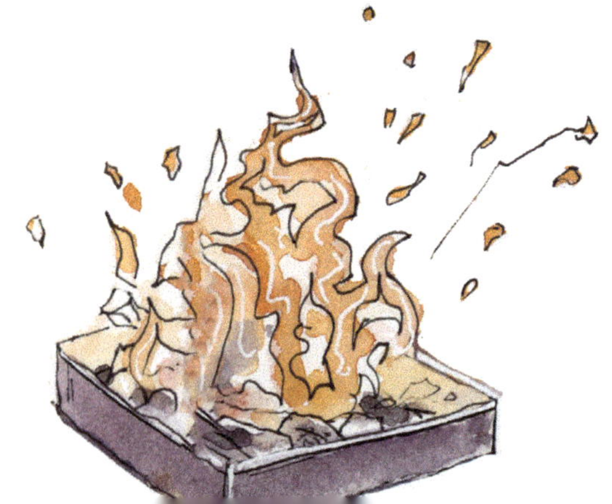

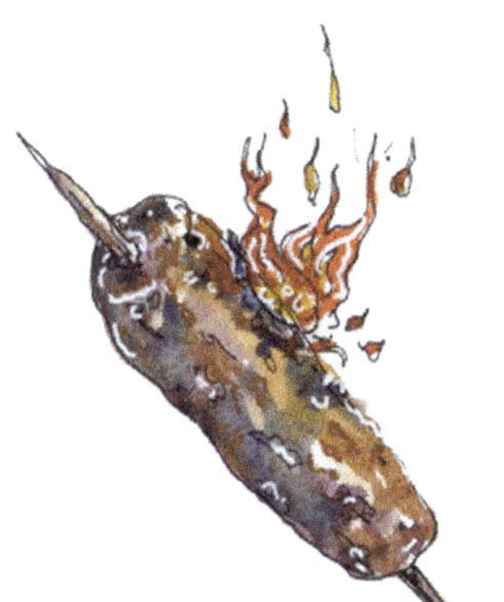

We were able to disrupt the intended order and outwit Mother Nature; we could now extend our days, buying ourselves more time. It allowed us to innovate, which, in turn, brought us increased comfort and convenience. But with this dominion there came the price of a separateness from the outdoors, without access to fresh air, to green space, and room for our bodies and minds to recalibrate. Like a thief in the night, 'man-made' slowly began to rob us of our health.

Needless to say, dinner that night, was in the woods. We threw some food and our trusty portable fire pan into a bag and hiked off into the forest under the cover of darkness. High in the hills, a fire leapt into life as the children foraged off into the blackness to fashion roasting sticks and suitable seats. Hours later we arrived back home feeling energised, re-fuelled and buzzing from our adventure!

It turns out that we don't need to run from, try to defeat or even fear nature. Rather, given the chance, it will strengthen your soul and its charm will exponentially grow ... like the love for your children.

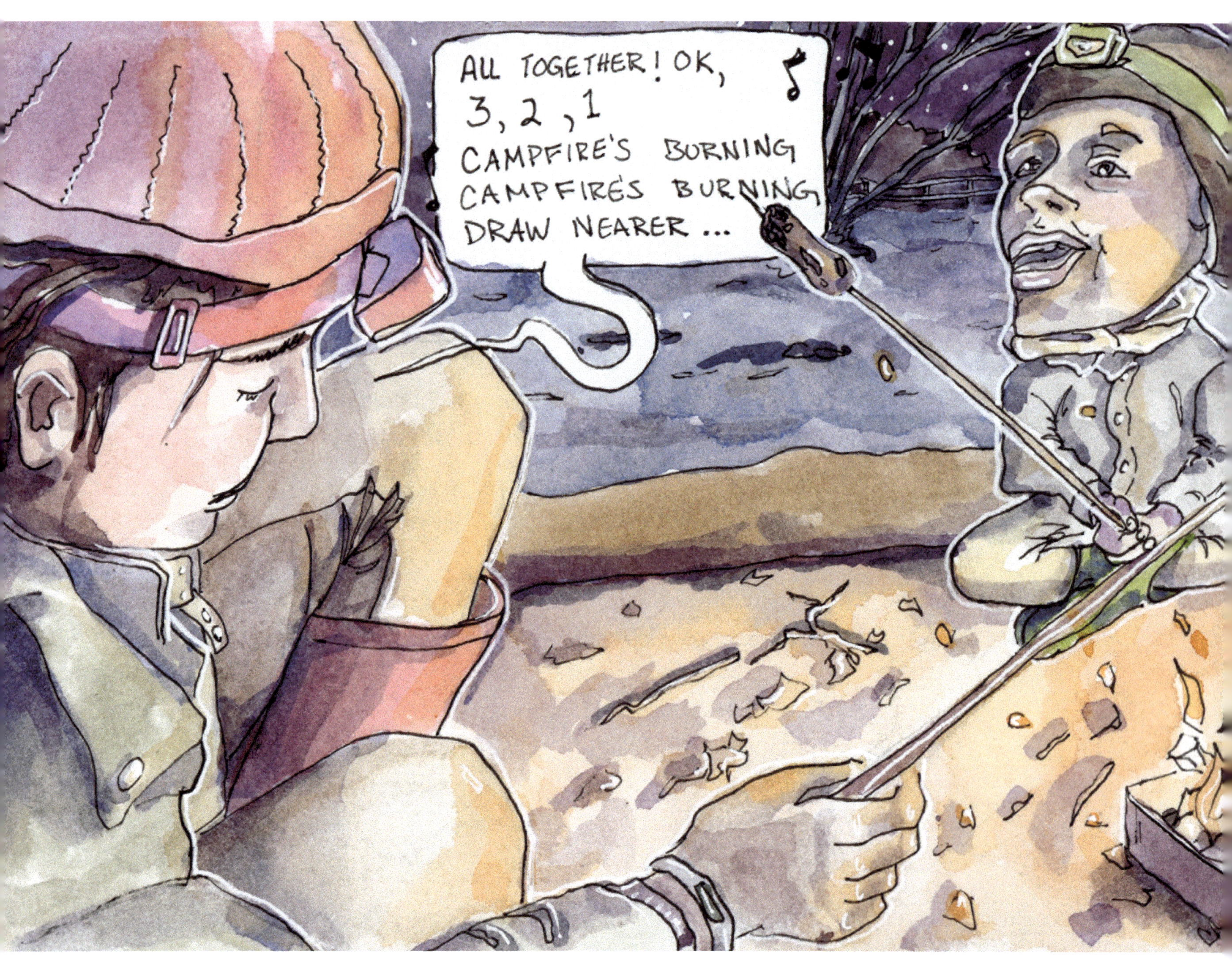

ALL TOGETHER! OK,
3, 2, 1
CAMPFIRE'S BURNING
CAMPFIRE'S BURNING
DRAW NEARER ...

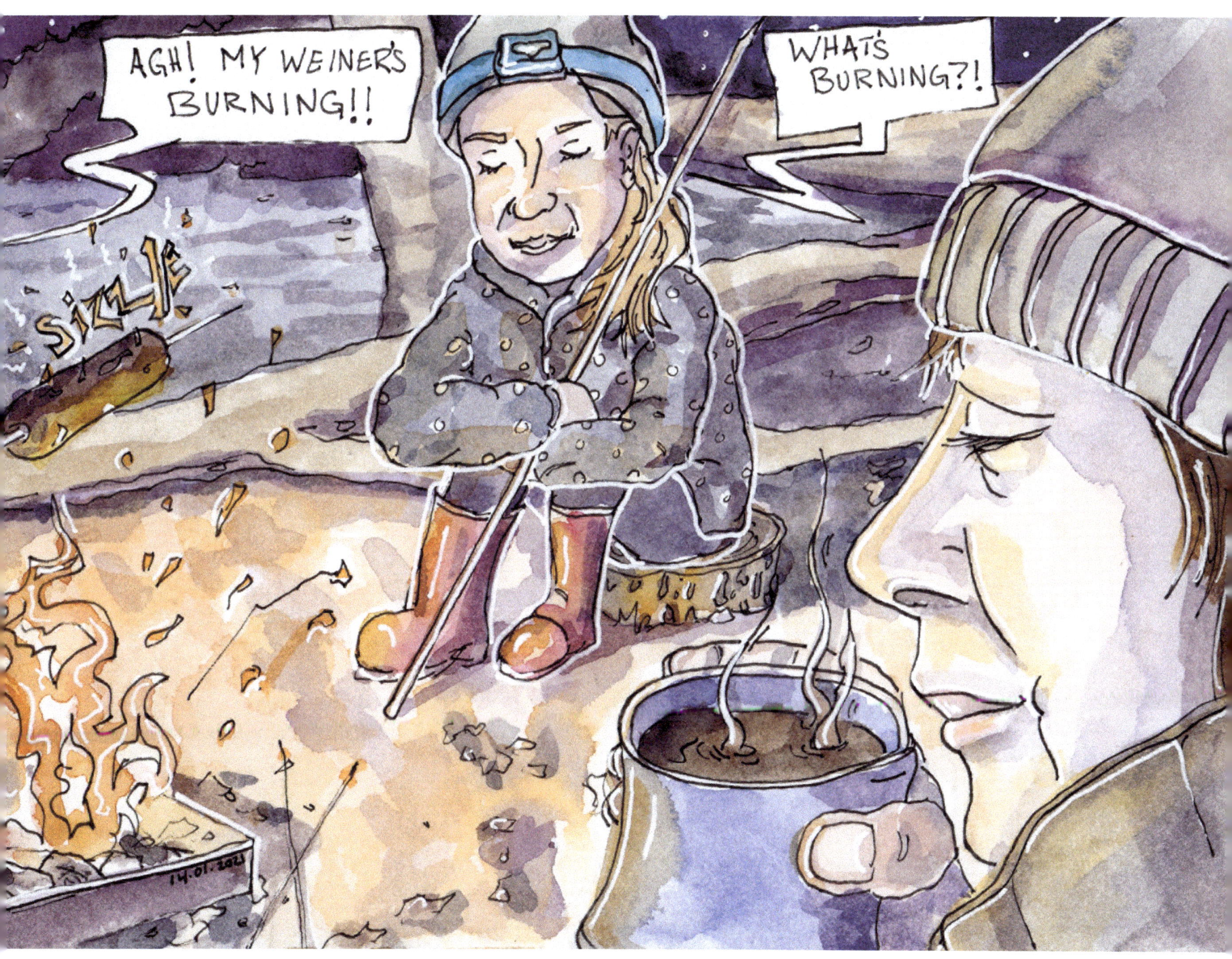

AGH! MY WEINER'S BURNING!!
WHAT'S BURNING?!
SIZZLE

CAPTAIN SIR TOM MOORE

AS FAR AS inspiring figures go, Captain Sir Tom Moore is at the top of the list.

From time to time, in my (mostly imagined) mid-life crisis, I have this recurring thought: am I too old? Too old to make a difference? Too old to make a significant mark? Has age punched the clock on this gaffer's timecard? It's all a bit melodramatic, I know, but I have this deep desire to know that my life has meaning. Then, bristling alongside these regular impervious musings of insignificance, is another thought: "It's not about what a person achieves, it's about who we become and how we serve people." For it is in those actions where we look outside of ourselves, and actively give to others, that we short-circuit a lonely navel-gazing existence and enable freedom and joy for others. There is something in the act of serving that leaves a permanent, indelible mark on the soul of both the giver and the receiver.

So, Captain Sir Tom, you are indeed an inspiration. Not simply because you walked 100 lengths of your garden and in doing so raised millions for NHS Charities Together, but because you determined to selflessly serve others. As a centenarian you bore the weight of a nation's anxiety on your forged shoulders. Seeing past perceived limitations, you brought us hope. It turns out that age is not a barrier. You have taught us about how to live with significance, one step at a time, and that "the sun will shine again, and the clouds will go away."

Thank you.

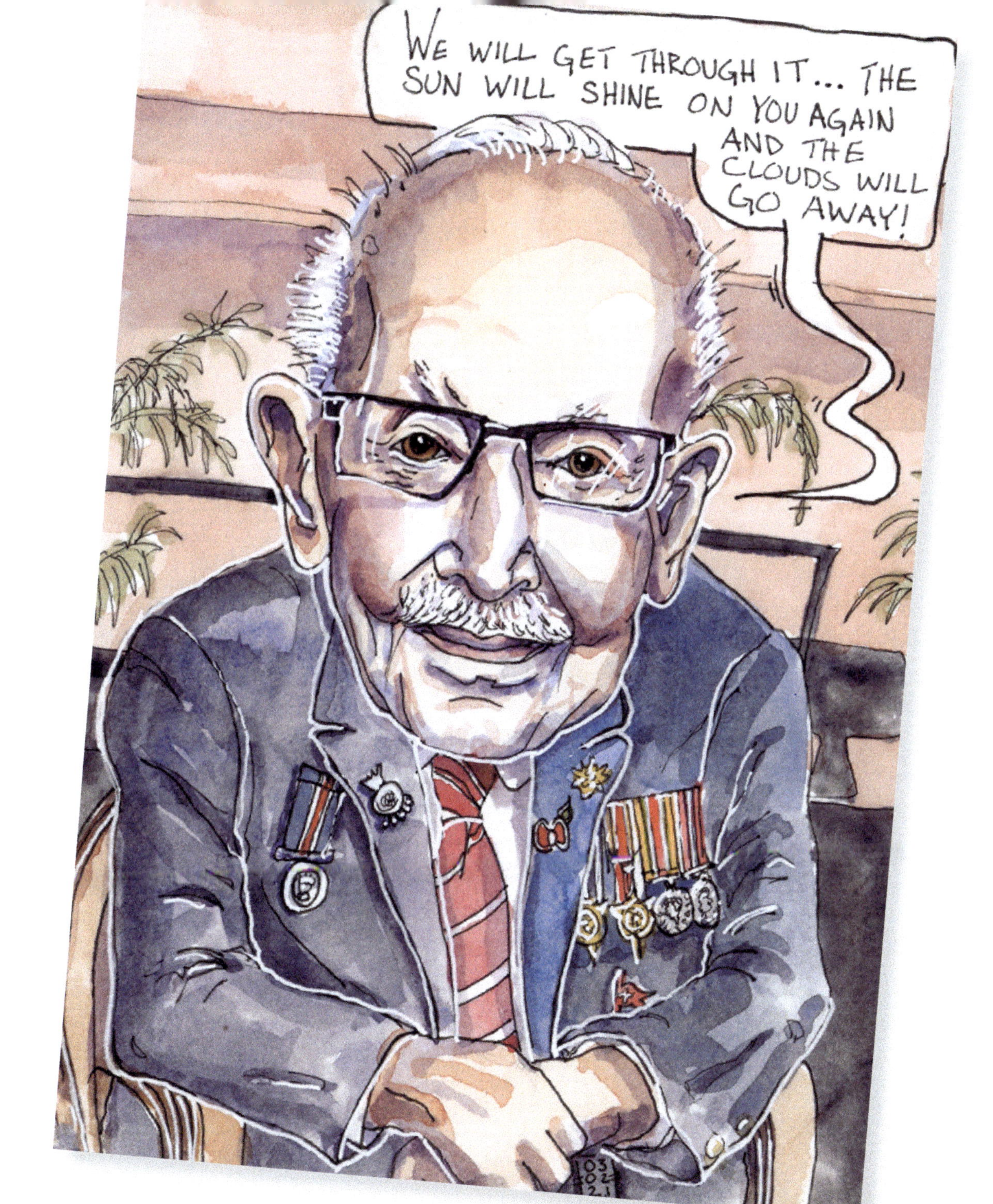

WE WILL GET THROUGH IT... THE
SUN WILL SHINE ON YOU AGAIN
AND THE
CLOUDS WILL
GO AWAY!

GETTING TO THE ROOT OF THE PROBLEM

'A MAN'S HOME is his castle', so, by virtue, the garden is his kingdom. My 'castle' lies atop of a hill, in the countryside overlooking a far-reaching valley. It sounds romantic. However, the plot has its fair share of quirks and challenges, which are further exacerbated by the previous owners' penchant for inspired additions. This idea was popular in the age of enlightenment when patrons would take part in the grand tour, collecting art and rare curiosities from around the Mediterranean. Then, bringing these rare antiquities back, their stately homes were adorned with these carefully curated masterpieces.

What our previous owners shared in enthusiasm with these early collectors, they lacked in taste. The cascading slopes of our garden were strewn with a random assortment of statues (Buddhas, pandas, toads and fairies), sundials, iridescent beads and even an ill-proportioned replica of David. However, the most flamboyant addition was their Pampas grass. Apparently, they had been wildly inspired on one of their trips to far flung Gran Canaria!

Pampas Grass is an invasive species in the UK with a knack for survival. Protecting their regal plums are long robust leaves that hide razor sharp barbs along their edges, their roots relentlessly grip the ground with their wiry tendrils. Their thirst for survival enables them to grow to ridiculously impressive proportions.

Fed up with the hours required to prune them back, I set out to remove these ostentatious plants, just as I had eradicated the mob of statues. In a moment of genius, I discovered what I imagined was the plants' Achilles heel! Each year, they regenerate, the old leaves die back leaving dried husks from which new shoots grow. Where there are dry leaves, there can surely be flames – and destruction. So, in an effort to simplify life, I carried out my coup. I waltzed down the drive to face my foe. Lighting a match, I dropped it into the heart of the brown gnarled beast. It was spectacular. As predicted the plant burst into an impressive fireball. Victory ... and smoke. Lots of smoke. Thick white smoke. The wind shifted, carrying it purposefully towards our unsuspecting cul-de-sac. Before long, the neighbourhood was shrouded in a thick white blanket. I ran to get the hosepipe. Perhaps if I dampened it slightly … !?

Then the people came. Heads popped up from all sides.

"I'm trying to dry my bed linen outside on the line!"

"You are not supposed to have bonfires now! Did you know it's bad for asthma?"

"The smell is filling my whole house!"

"My ex-husband used to do this type of thing all the time."

Needless to say, I was not popular, and had to subsequently work hard at patching up those damaged relationships. However, I felt satisfied that the pampas were eradicated; all that remained was a charred pile of ash. As I fantasised about clearing away the charred remains to make way for a simpler palette, I was horrified to find that, a mere week later, a plethora of green shoots were charging up through the blackened remains, making a surge for a new life!

In the end, I had to admit defeat. I called in the cavalry, hiring a digger to remove the deeply entrenched monsters.

Having gone through this process, I can now see the deep parallel with my own life. The habits accumulated over a lifetime are deeply rooted; my peacocking 'achievements' and vain efforts sitting awkwardly on the landscape of my history, proudly waving but incongruous to a sense of harmony. It is difficult to eradicate these parts that grow to overshadow the simplicity and goodness. Now that I have had time to breathe, I can see that trying to prune back these things with holidays, accumulating 'stuff' and striving toward bigger ambition are all a bit like a wayward traveller aimlessly gathering a hodgepodge of antiquities. The rat race overshadows. But when you take control and remove those things, from the roots, clearing away all that distracts, you are left with clarity. It turns out that there is real power in simplicity; it yields clarity, joy and peace. It took a heart attack to uproot my life. Now with the plumage gone, I can see a way forward, life recalibrated to honour the time I have been given here on earth.

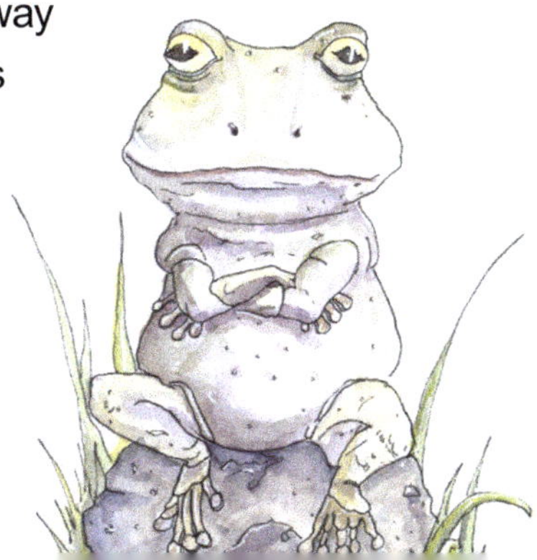

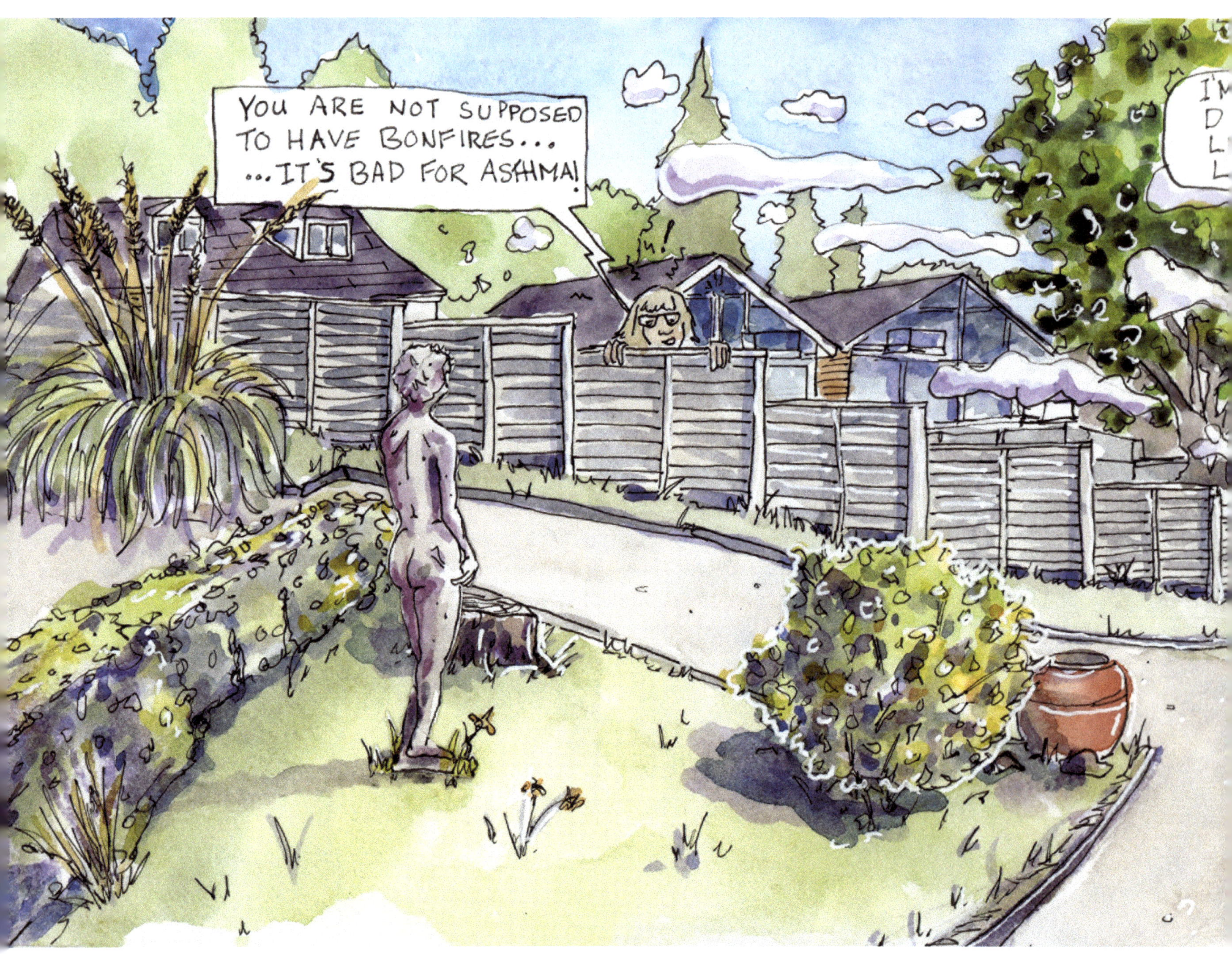

YOU ARE NOT SUPPOSED TO HAVE BONFIRES... ...IT'S BAD FOR ASHMA!
I'M
D
L L

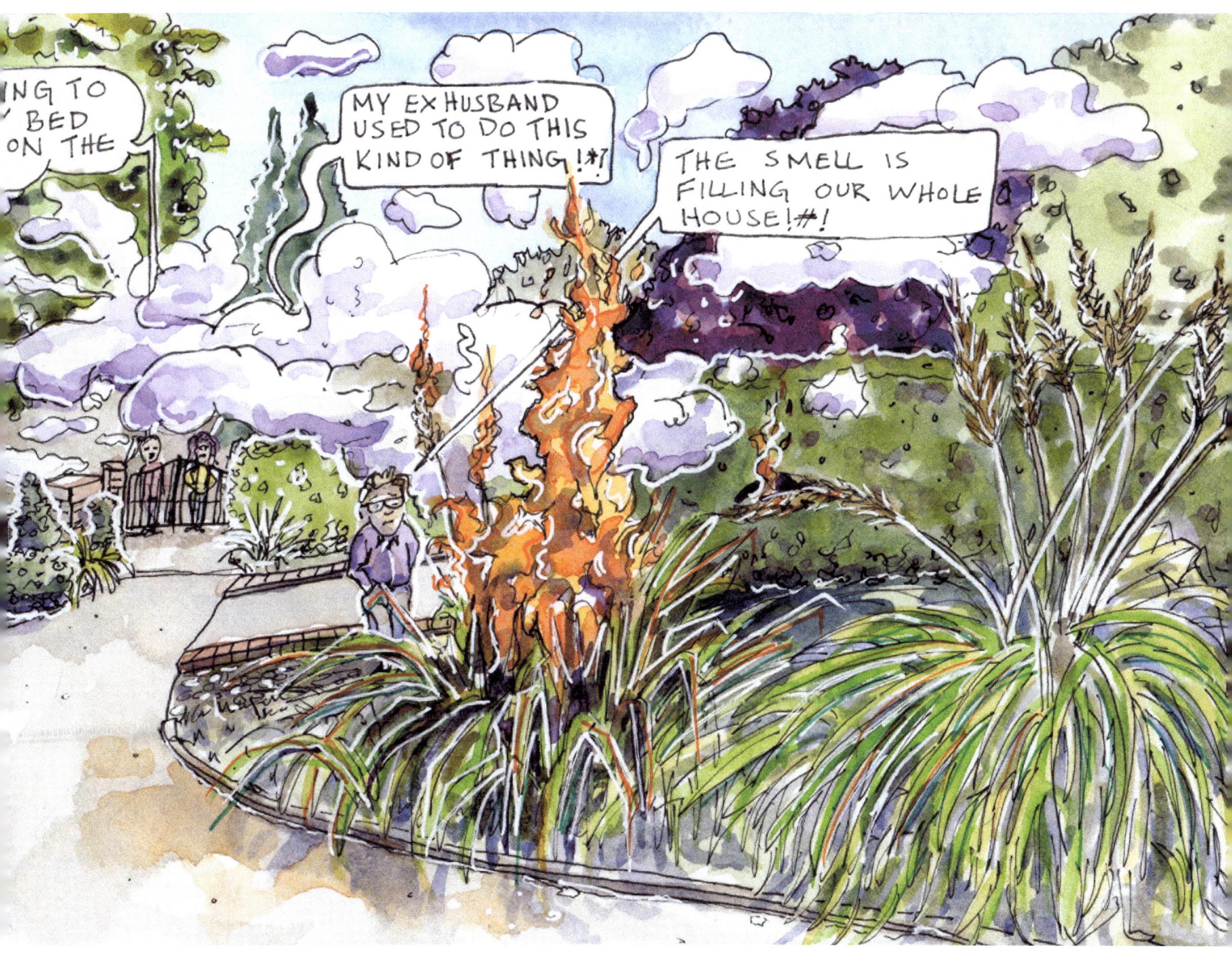

ING TO
BED
ON THE
MY EX HUSBAND USED TO DO THIS KIND OF THING !*?
THE SMELL IS FILLING OUR WHOLE HOUSE!#!

A TALE OF TWO PANS

HORROR! For the first time in my life, I was to be shackled!

I had just been whisked into the emergency room by the paramedics. Still in denial of what could possibly have happened, I sat, wide-eyed as the nurse swiftly took my bloods and conducted a small battery of tests. I was left to think like an errant schoolboy until the doctor finally arrived, striding into my cubicle, slightly distracted but with a suitable look of concern on his face. He closed the door, sat down at his computer and, after heavily pecking at his keyboard for a minute, looked up and dryly pronounced, "Based on the markers in your blood and your blood pressure, which was extraordinarily high, you have had a heart attack, likely a series of heart attacks."

That moment is permanently burnt into my memory. The proclamation was shrouded by disbelief as a million different thoughts ran through my mind. "Are you sure? What does this mean? I have so much work to do! Can I go home now? Should I go home now? The lights are so bright! My will! It's out of date. Quick! Find a bit of paper!"

Then, as though it were as natural as crocs on a doctor, he casually added, "You will now be on medication for the rest of your life."

If the impact of the previous moment had left me with questions, this statement hit me like a wrecking ball and sent me reeling. In that instant, it felt as if my entire way of life would be shackled. The thought of having to take medication religiously each day for the rest of my life seemed to be a placard of limitation, daily highlighting my weakness and preventing the freedom I so dearly love. "No, no, no," I lamented, "only my grandparents, the elderly, have to take medication daily!" This life sentence seemed more of a blow than the heart attack itself.

Days later, after having been released from the hospital, my wife, sensing that I was still struggling with the noose of taking a daily cocktail of eight different tablets, thought she would soften the impact by buying me a pill dispenser. It was a 'cheerful' rainbow-coloured pan neatly organised into the seven daily pockets. But the fact is, there is no disguising the truth; "You can dress a monkey in silk, but it is still a monkey."

Throughout this life-changing process, I have had another pan at my side, nearly daily. Curiously though, these tethers have been comforting, grounding, even inspiring. Also organised into a rainbow of colours, my watercolour pan has been a lifeline. In fact, it has brought a sense of purpose and optimism, it has allowed me to 'see' what I couldn't before, and uniquely observe the beauty in the world around me. Joy.

It turns out, that shackles can hold you still enough to see freedom.

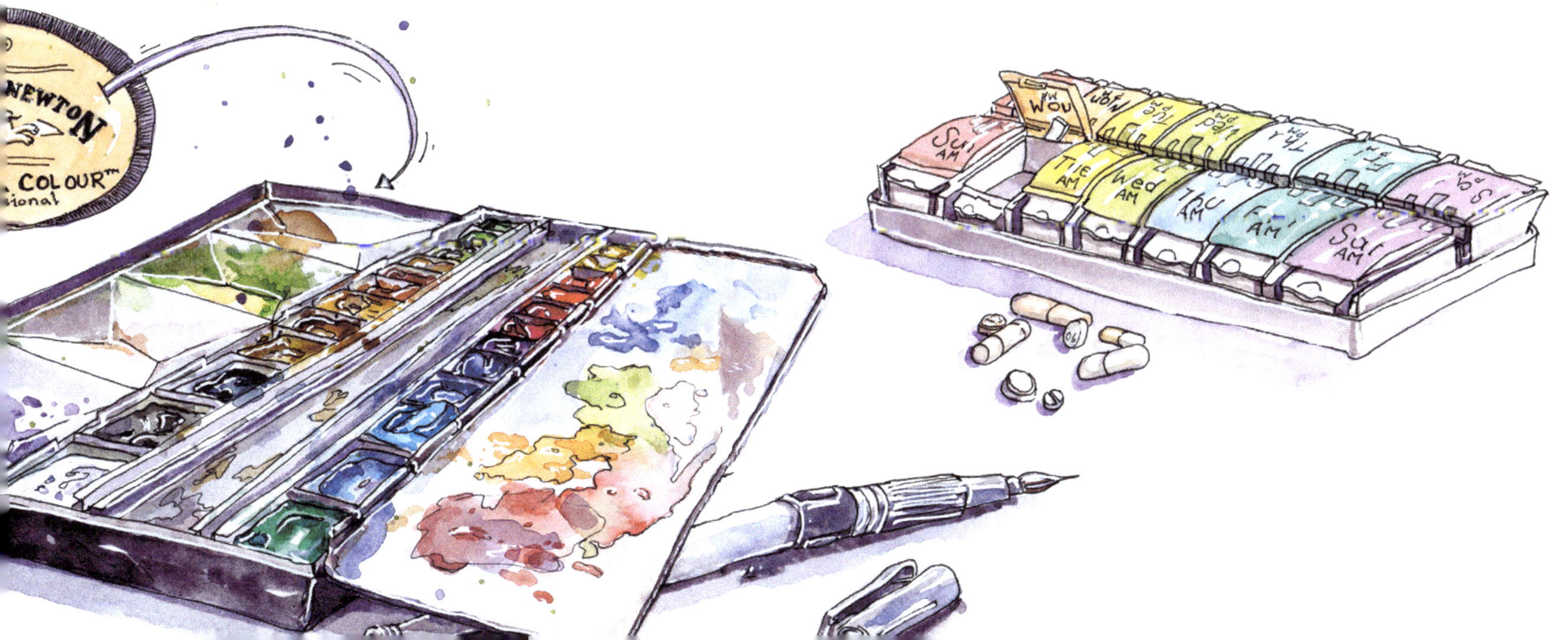

Renewal

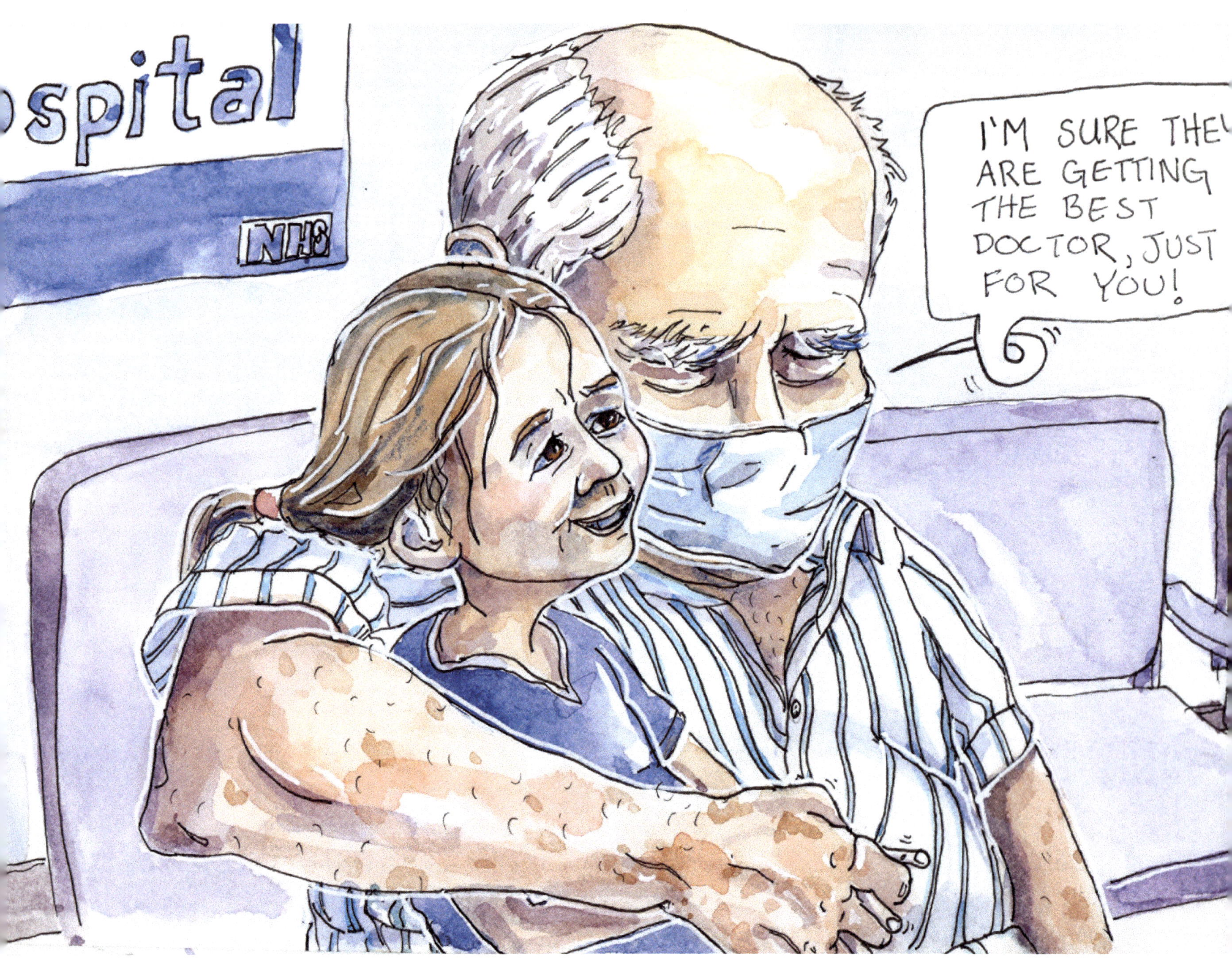
ospital
NHS
I'M SURE THEY
ARE GETTING
THE BEST
DOCTOR, JUST
FOR YOU!

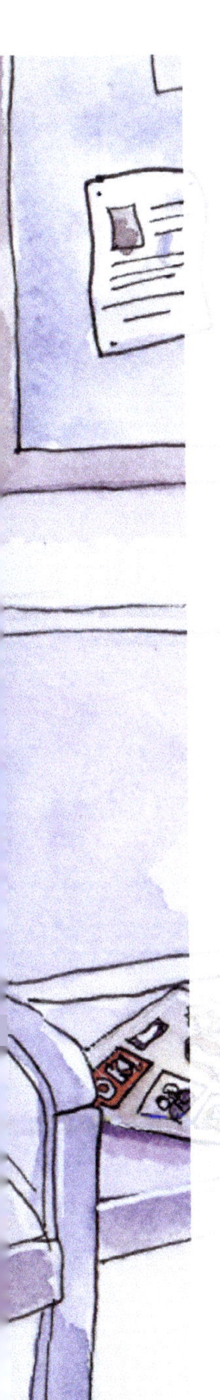

HOLDING HANDS

WHEN WAS THE LAST TIME your hand was held by someone's bigger than yours?
I recently trundled down to my local clinic for a little medical top-up. There has been a definite increase in the frequency of these sorts of visits post heart attack. While I sat in the lobby, avoiding the lure of my phone and consciously trying to be more present, I spotted what appeared to be a grandfather with his granddaughter. Sitting there in the melee of ailing patients, each assigned to a soulless metal chair and lined up like military recruits, the young girl looked around wide-eyed and clearly overwhelmed. These sterile institutions are rarely welcoming. Instinctively she pressed her weight into her granddad's warm flannel shirt. Sensing the need for security, he gently slipped his big leathery hand around hers and gave it a squeeze. In that moment her anxiety melted away, and a small smile appeared in the corners of her mouth. I, too, melted. The unforced smile on my face an endorsement of that powerful act. I vividly remember, as a young boy, holding my own grandfather's hand, my palms dwarfed by his powerful yet gentle grip. Comfort.

Even now, with nearly half a century of life under my belt, I still feel the reassurance of that act; the vulnerability of humanity given security. As my mind flooded with warm endorphins, I suddenly had an unexpected thought, "When was the last time my hand had been held by someone's bigger than my own?" It had been a very long time. My heart sunk in self-pity as I fruitlessly searched the caverns of my mind.

Then, after a few moments of emptiness, another thought arrived. It was small, then quickly grew. "It needn't come to me." My heart pulsed. "I can be that man. I can offer that warm protective grasp for those in my life." I could feel a visceral flutter of joy in my chest and a sense of renewed mission!

Revelations like these seem to be strange new occurrences, arriving as a result of having damaged my own heart. I now feel more compassionate, as though the event has removed the scales of malice and revived a sense of purpose.

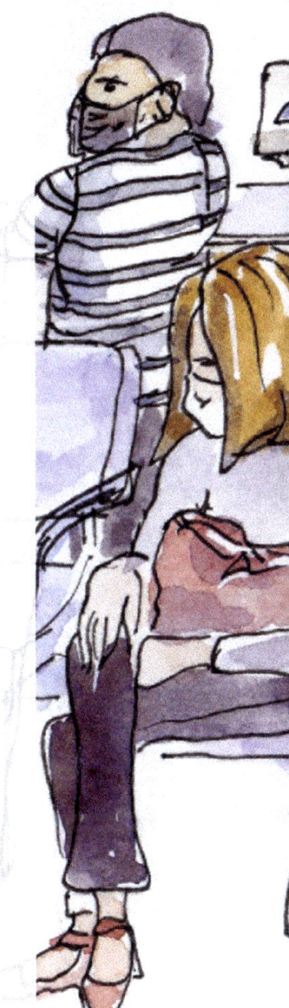

RECOVERY, COURTESY OF THE MAGIC PILL

IF YOU SEE IT offered, know that it does not exist. Tantalised by an apothecary of advertised miracle cures, I have been tempted and have tried. I have been on the lookout for 'a pill' that will undo all the wrongs I have imposed on my body over the past four and half decades.

Alas, there is no pill but, as with a hearty homemade soup, I am realising that renewal requires a finely tested concoction of carefully chosen ingredients. To belabour the metaphor, in the kitchen of life, I have stumbled upon what might just be the secret recipe. For starters, the outdoors is essential; its power to connect us to natural rhythms and its ability to draw us back to a sense of balance is extraordinary. The Norwegians have a term for this, it is called friluftsliv, or 'free air life'. It elevates the human desire for uplifting experiences while underscoring the need for happiness and mental health. It's as though our soul is reminded that we are part of something that is much bigger than ourselves.

I was recently camping in the forest. Although the mercury had dropped, the tent was cosy. The moon was nearly full, illuminating the sentient woodland, and a symphony of sounds danced through the ambient night. Curiosity and wonder awoke.

On the topic of sleep, mine has recently (intentionally) increased. I have garnered a regular rhythm of sleep that has dramatically brought my average up to the 8.5-hour mark. This shift, from an anaemic six hours per night, has done wonders to allow my body to heal and repair. True physical restoration.

When I was a boy, I would visit my grandparents from the 'old country'. Beneath a carefully placed painting reminding us to give thanks, my sister and I would be served porridge with prunes and brown sugar for breakfast. "It is essential for a good day," we were told. Years later I have rediscovered porridge. Inspired by early pioneers, I have come to enjoy my daily gruel, with a few enhancements of course – blueberries, banana, almond butter, cacao nibs and maple syrup – a breakfast of champions! And, if I'm on the go, the overnight variety in a mason jar is a nice alternative.

And my latest experiments have been in the exploration of a cleaner diet. Veganuary was a revelation. For a lifetime, I bought into the belief that a meal is not really a meal without carnivorous detailing. But, as it turns out, a plant-based diet, carefully curated can be quite invigorating, and tasty!

I feel uncannily well.

Ultimately, though, the proof of all this experimentation has been in the science (the metric that the world endorses). My wife lovingly bought me a blood pressure monitor. After regularly measuring my blood pressure, I have seen my levels approaching what medical professionals would call 'ideal'. So no, there is no miracle pill, certainly nothing particularly modern or jazzy, just a return to a collection of age-old simple practices.

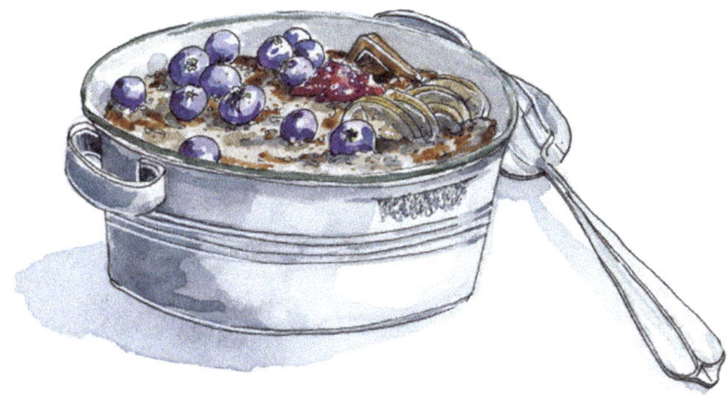

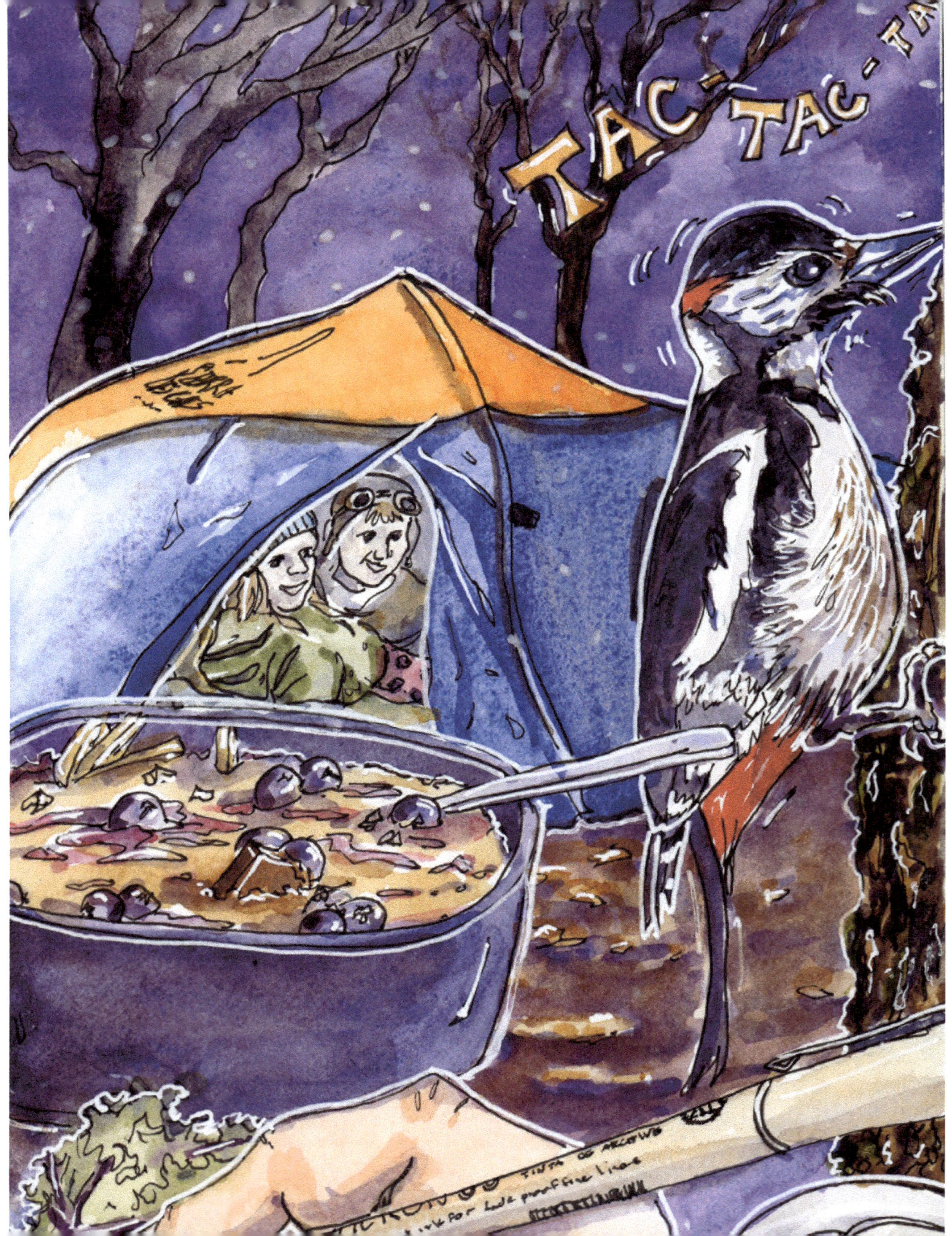
TAC-TAC-TA

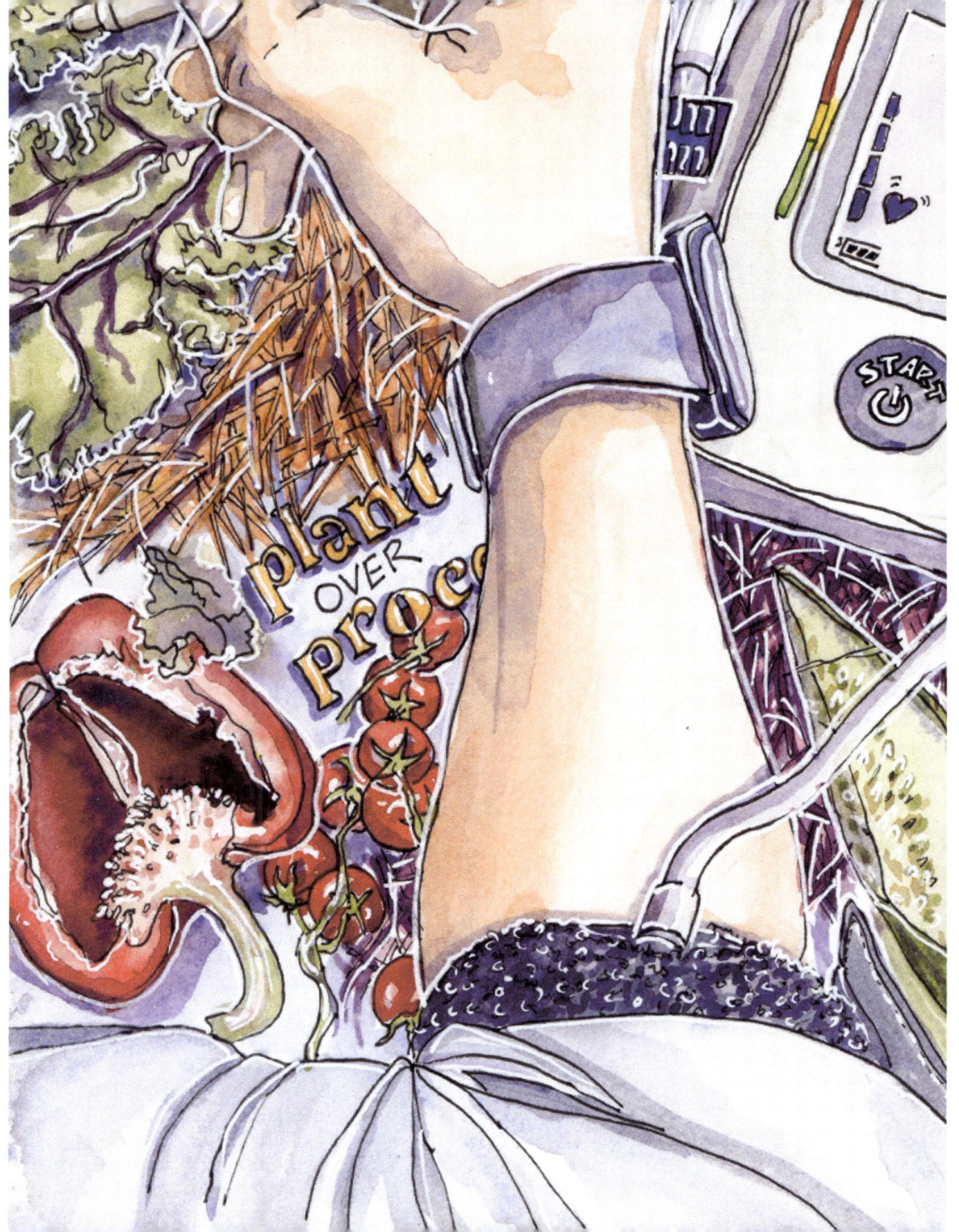

START
plant
OVER
proc

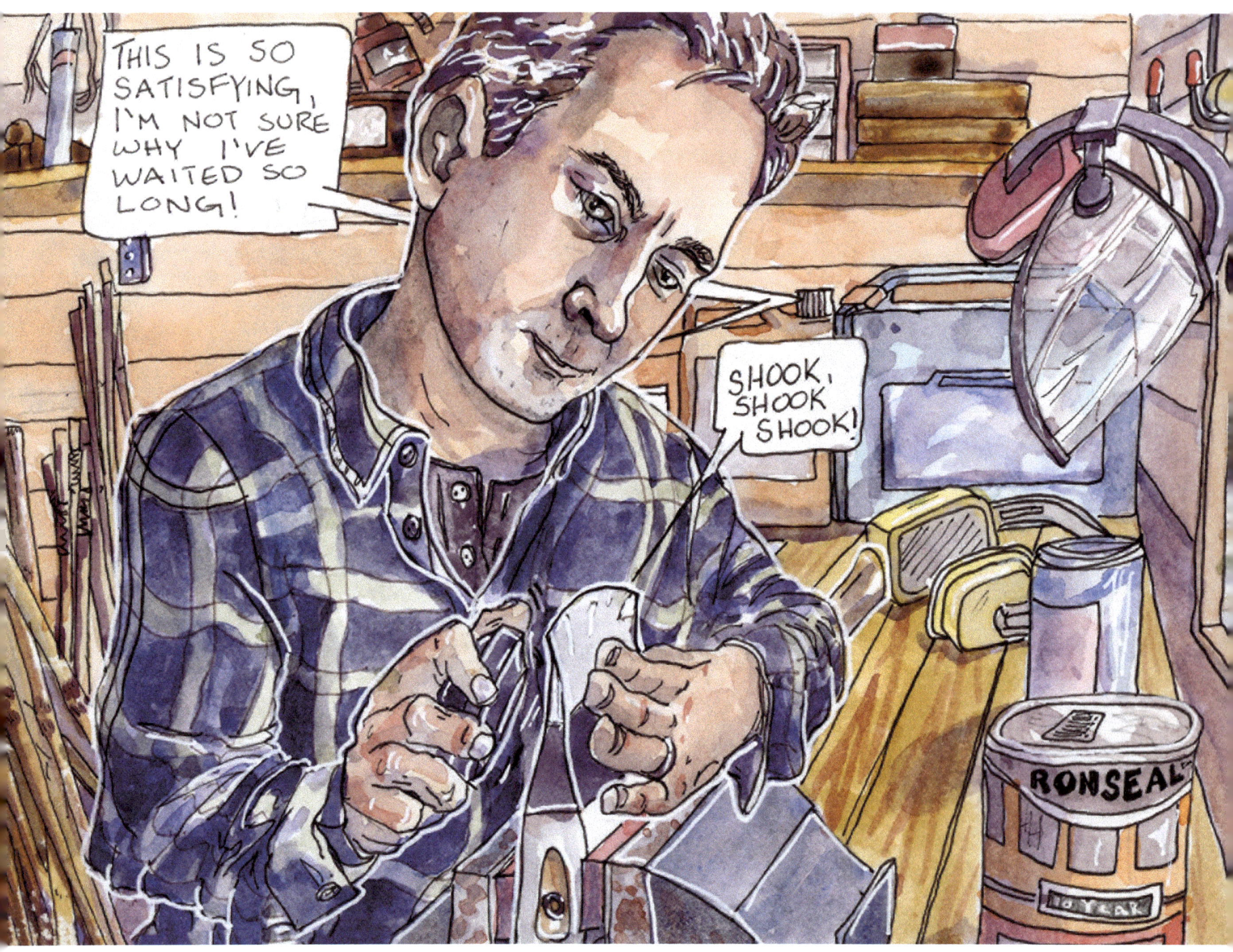

THIS IS SO SATISFYING, I'M NOT SURE WHY I'VE WAITED SO LONG!
SHOOK, SHOOK SHOOK!
RONSEAL
10 YEAR

AN AXE TO GRIND

I RECENTLY received a rather handsome axe from my wife. I had been pining after one for quite some time and was after that pure rush of dopamine that accompanies the fell swoop of an axe through an unsuspecting log on a crisp morning.

Upon opening the neatly wrapped package, I was not disappointed. The strong ash handle, beautifully formed and perfectly tooled, led to a soft leather sheath surrounding the head. With great excitement I released the blade from its protective case. In an instant, the forged steel glimmered as it caught the morning light streaming through the window. My eyes widened; I imagined the fine work that I could do with this magnificent tool. A good friend of mine, who takes the act of sharpening very seriously, measures the readiness of a cutting edge by its ability to delicately shave off a patch of arm hair. I couldn't resist. Surely this blade would rival that of a samurai sword! My thumb made its way to the blade and gingerly stroked the edge. To my horror it was blunt; the cutting edge was as flat as a 2 pence piece worn by time in a pocket.

Resolutely, I immediately set to work learning the art of sharpening. It would take quite some work to bring the under-loved steel to a finely tuned blade. I invested in the necessary equipment and, when it arrived, I made my way to the shed. Tightly clamping the axe in a vice, I began to work the steel. Initially with a rasp, working the blade to some semblance of a point, then with my new sharpening stone I spent the better part of the next two hours refining the edge. My shoulder was sore but the gentle circular strokes, evenly balanced on both sides, gradually wore away the surplus steel which was now blackening my fingers. Finally, a lethal edge emerged.

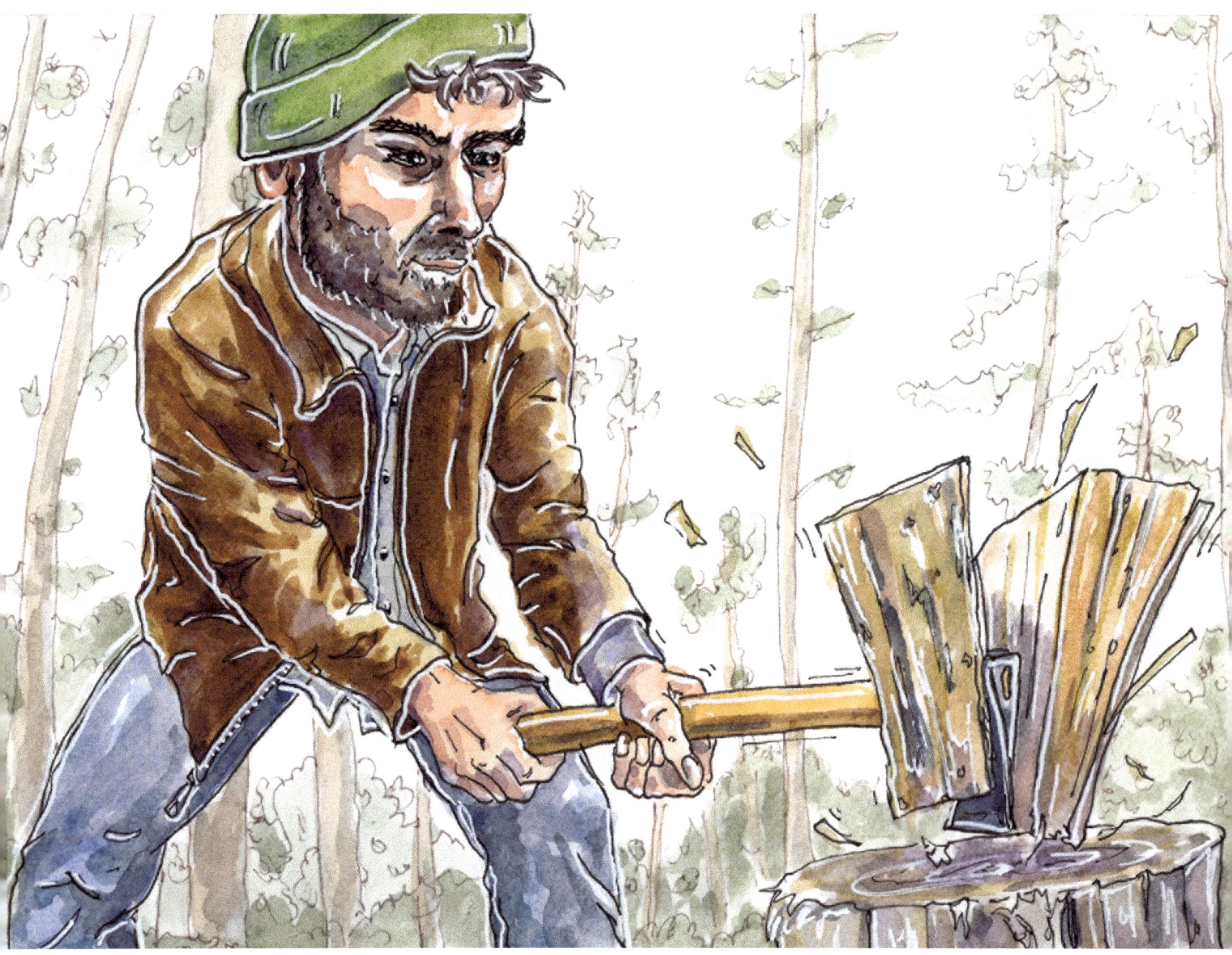

It was sharp. Very sharp. The hair test – a success! But now the real test, a log. Summoning an unsuspecting bolt of beech, I perched it on a chopping block. Feeling the need to make an impact I took a mighty swing. Feeling a ripple of power explode up from my hips, through my torso, shoulders and finally into my hands, the blade obliterated the log in one clean cut! Like a hot knife through soft butter, it was a success! I could feel my heart surge with joy.

I am discovering that life is a bit like an axe. It can be sharp and purposeful, but if left unattended or misused it becomes blunt and ineffective; the force then needed to do anything is great. So, how do you get to the point where your effectiveness feels effortless? It starts, I am learning, with a deep look at the tool itself. Discover your God-given superpower, the spaces in your life that feel effortless and bring great joy. Then, invest in the tools that will help you grow in those areas and grind. Not the exhausting grind but the gritty, get lost in the task grind, the kind that despite the intense focus, feels like effortless joy.

So, for the second time in recent months, I am sharpening an 'axe', working on bringing my life to a razor-sharp point. I recently read a short musing from an old woodsman, who noted that, when taken care of, a good axe lasts a lifetime and even leaves its mark on the next generation.

Nice.

THE BEAUTIFUL VESSEL – A LESSON IN KINTSUKUROI

I HAVE NEVER REALLY liked the idea of cosmetic surgery. It is a fight against nature, and in that duel, you are bound to lose because, in the end, nature always wins. But I would be lying if I told you that I had not entertained the idea of getting a few replacement parts – just the essentials, of course, to help with the ageing process. My back is pretty dodgy, so I'd have a few new vertebrae (something in titanium appeals) and a new heart, perhaps one designed for a world-class ironman athlete. Out with the old, in with the new!

Despite our mortal desires, life has a way of surprising us with unexpected twists. In this case, I stumbled across an idea. A revelation. It was a concept that would transform my small, insular, self-pitying notion that 'new is better'. In the fifteenth century, the Japanese art of kintsukuroi (golden repair) emerged. It involves the restoration of shattered ceramics with urushi lacquer and powdered metal, most commonly gold. The central idea of kintsukuroi is that an object is made more beautiful by its history, and that when it is broken through time and usage, it amasses a story. The term for this marvellous philosophy is wabi-sabi, which translates as finding beauty in that which is imperfect, incomplete, impermanent, and marked by time. Under the skilled hands of the artist, a broken ceramic is transformed, through careful attention, into something more beautiful than it was before.

When I look on at seasoned sailors and hardened adventurers, their hair bleached, faces windblown and furrowed by the unrelenting elements, and hands calloused rough from a lifetime of struggle, I see beauty, and I look on in awe and admiration. They have earned their scars, and their stories bear testament to a life well lived. Then, by comparison, I look at my broken heart – a less than perfect, shattered vessel damaged by a lifetime of abuse. It seems impossible to find any beauty there. And yet, upon closer inspection, I am very much alive, optimistically walking the road of recovery having been given a chance to recalibrate life with a fresh perspective.

The skilled hands of many 'artists' have been at work on me – doctors, family, friends and pastors. They have rescued my arteries and, surprisingly, something much deeper, a part of my soul. It turns out that I am in the midst of a great adventure. My story has become much more beautiful as a result of my brokenness.

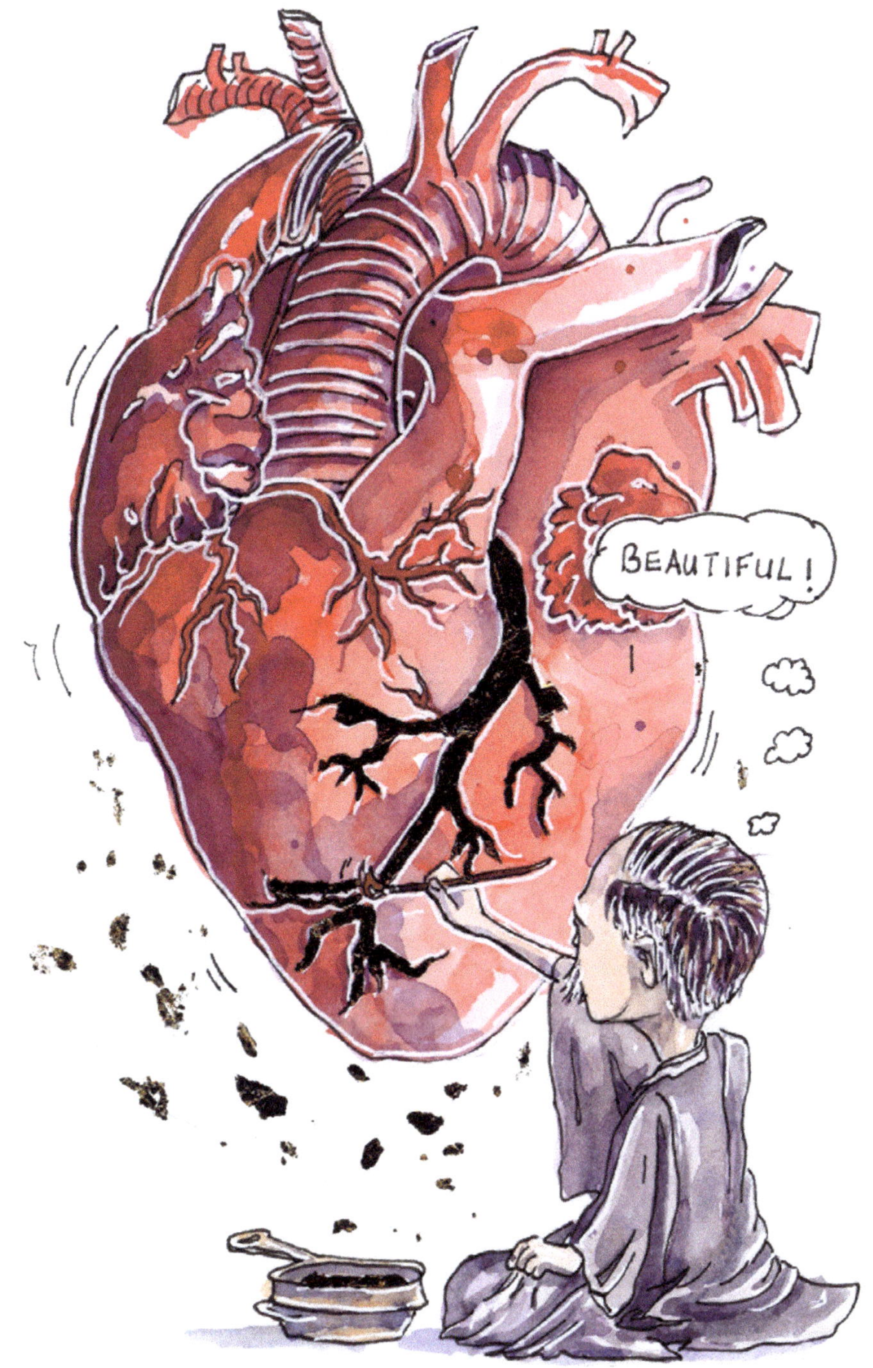
BEAUTIFUL!

A TURQUOISE BLUR

ON A PARTICULARLY picturesque day, I had decided to take a stroll through my local park. It was one of those perfect days, the kind that magnetically draws people out of their routines with promises of restoration and hope. All of humanity was out basking. Some prostrate in the lush green grass, others gently meandering along carefully edged paths, while others, mostly children, energetically buzzed around savouring the freedom.

In an unexpected moment my peripheral radar picked up a potentially concerning object careering toward me. Instinctually, I leapt aside in an impulsive, and somewhat awkward, jig. The movement, as it turns out, was justified, for in that instant, a young dandy on his bike roared by in a turquoise blur. He was clearly embroiled in a marvellous (largely imagined) escapade. His heroism was underscored by his homemade cardboard flames roaring out from his handcrafted exhaust. As his chiselled grin evaporated into the distance, a dapper gentleman came into focus. He was sitting on a park bench neatly tucked behind a newspaper. As I looked on at his still frame, his youth and dynamism a distant memory, I wondered, at what point he had stopped playing? Then, a surprising and equally nebulous question crept into my mind. When did I stop playing? I couldn't help but think that there must be a connection between that point and when my heart started to suffer ill effects?

Shedding some light on the issue of play is science, which has grappled with this topic and has proven a multitude of benefits like reduced stress, improved creativity, soaring joy and sharpened connection to others. However, in my mind, the most poignant advantage is play's ability to improve vitality and our resistance to disease.

George Bernard Shaw once said, "We don't stop playing because we grow old; we grow old because we stop playing." So, with that truth in mind, it is my mission to reengage with play. On my bucket list: a return to games nights; more time in the natural world; a trip to the joke shop; building a lightsabre; and, especially, more time in far-flung adventures with kids.

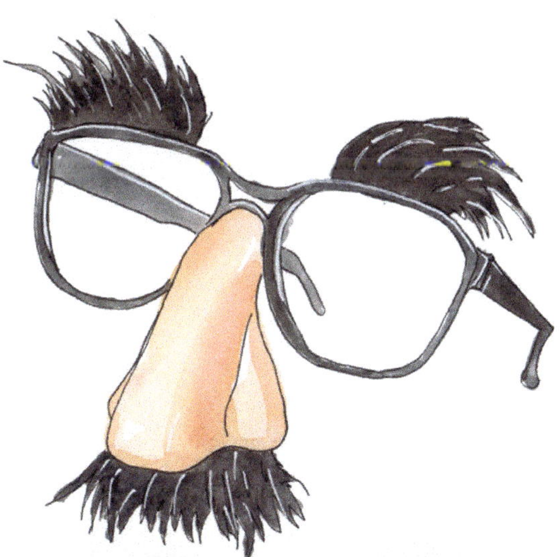

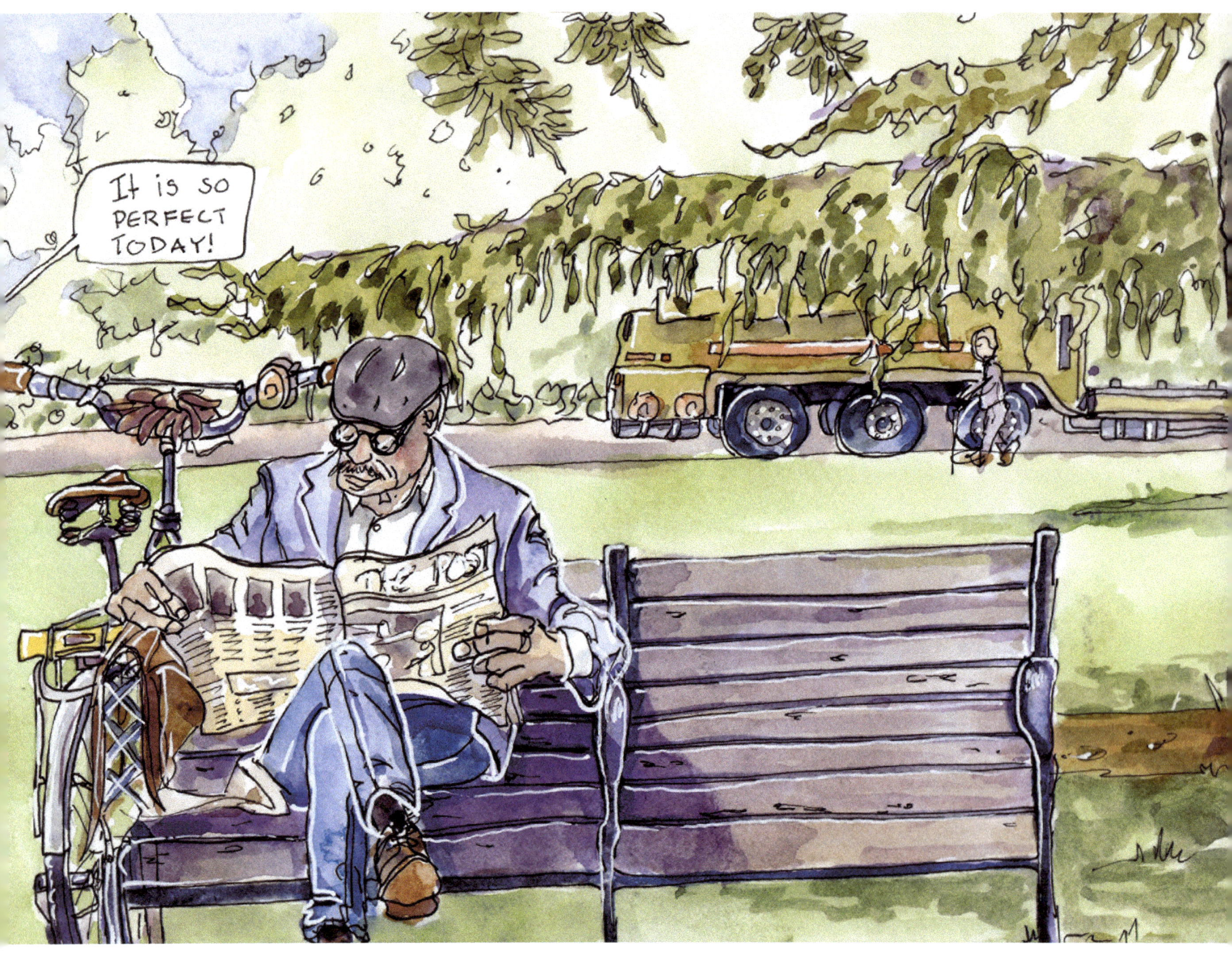

It is so perfect today!

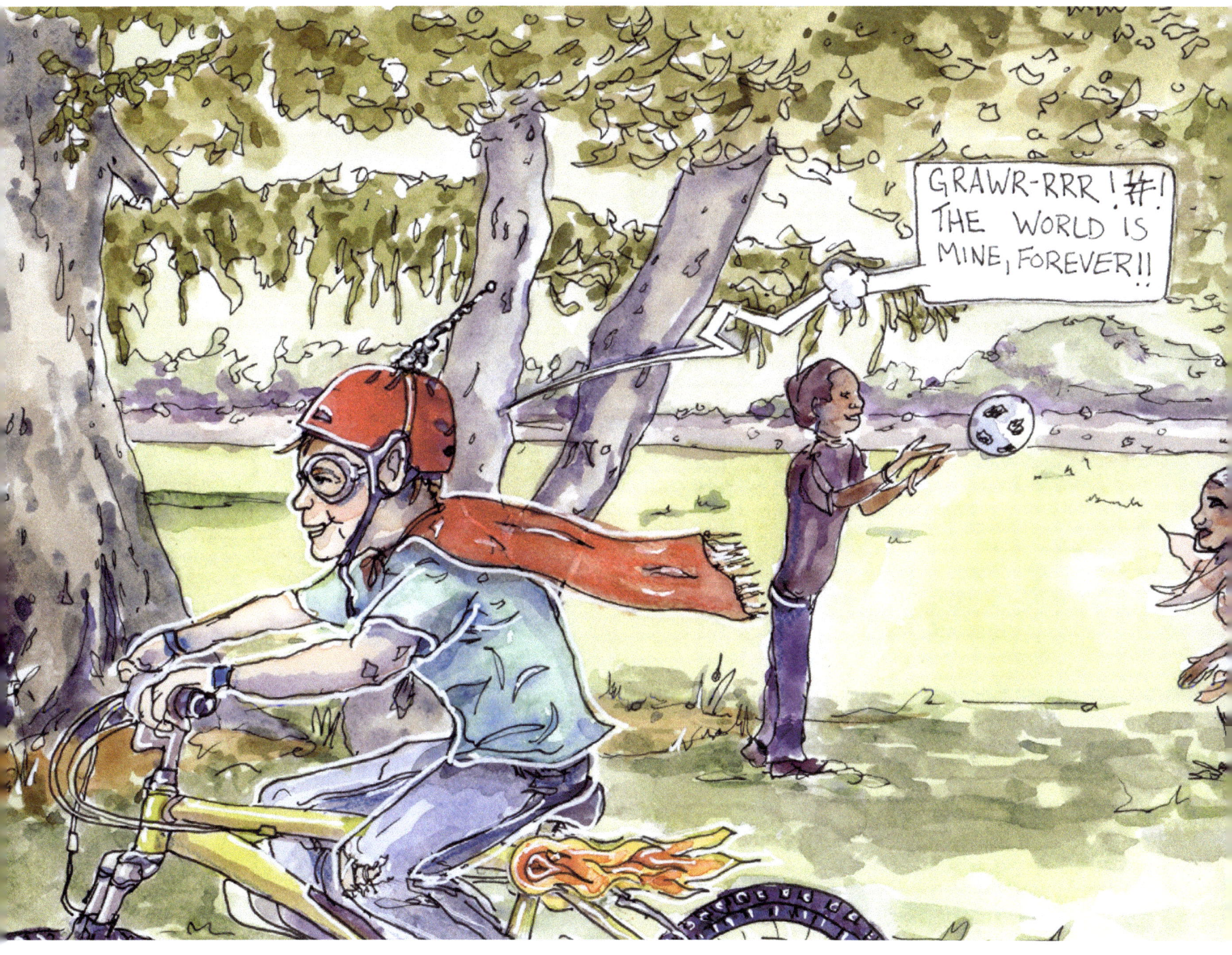

GRAWR-RRR ! #! THE WORLD IS MINE, FOREVER!!

JEAN'S TUNE-UP

SUMMER HAD ARRIVED in its full glory. The warm sunshine evaporating the
accumulated rain from the month prior. It was very welcome, but it revealed a
weakness – my car's air-conditioning had failed. I called up my local garage and
arranged for a quick tune-up. I arrived for my scheduled appointment and was
greeted by an upbeat, well-greased mechanic who told me that it would take a couple
of hours to mend the problem. So, I left and wondered down the country lane to explore
the locale. As I whimsically strolled along the leafy road admiring spring' artwork, I spotted a
cottage with a neat yellow door and a perfectly quaint flower garden. This was Jean's house. I had
heard about this local heroine. Exponentially inspiring, at 98 years of age she, apparently, still did
yoga, was a voracious artist and until last year, drove a cherry-red sportscar. Mustering my courage,
I decided to seize the opportunity and pop in. As I rounded the manicured hedge, the fullness of
her old cottage came into view. On a ladder balanced a tattooed handyman carefully cleaning the
windows and below, inspecting the work, was the frame of a slight, white-haired lady. I suddenly
felt very self-conscious, realising that I was awkwardly standing on her pea shingle drive staring
at her. I considered whether I should quickly turn and leave. But in that moment, she turned and
spotted me, like a rogue pheasant sniffed out by a gun dog. Surprised, and very suspicious, she
eyed me up and down, then, in a frightfully posh voice and with an air of authority said, "Hello, may
I help you?"

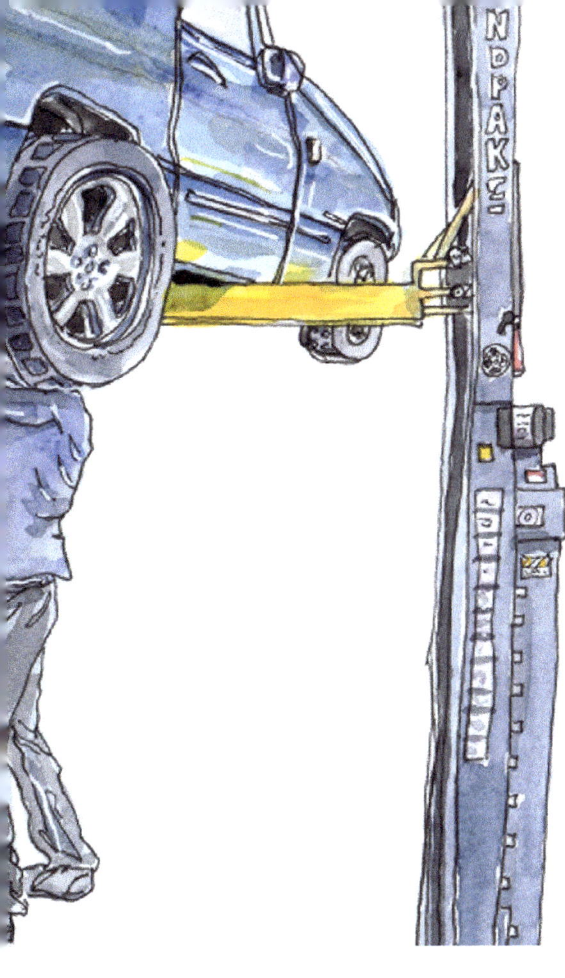

I was now committed. Feeling like an errant schoolboy I awkwardly stumbled over my introduction and blurted out my safety card, "I am Ian and Anji's son-in-law." There was a delicate moment of silence where her piercing grey eyes penetrated deep into my soul. Then, I saw it. Her suspicious stare melted away to reveal the very attribute that had been heralded in legend; it was a deep warmth that consumed every inch of her face, a warmth that emanated a whole-hearted welcome. What succeeded was a sumptuous conversation about life, art and connection ... and octopus neurology. "Aren't they just marvellous creatures, Jeff?" she exclaimed. She seemed to embody every good quality in humanity: curiosity, warmth, ingenuity and authenticity. As I left the impromptu meeting that afternoon, I felt inspired and lighter. A sense of hope filled the chasms of my searching heart, for I had discovered that a life well lived, one with longevity, is one that sees opportunity in the everyday and embraces it with warmth. That day the trajectory of my life was altered slightly by a chance collision with Jean. A metaphorical tune-up to accompany that of my ageing vehicle.

Postscript:
Before I left, Jean graciously thanked me for my visit, then asked for my number. "I promise I will not be a nuisance," she reassured me. Although that was the furthest thing from my mind, I was reminded of the importance of generations. We all have something to give and, if you allow it, sharing can lead to a rich and satisfying life. We have a great responsibility to take care of one another.

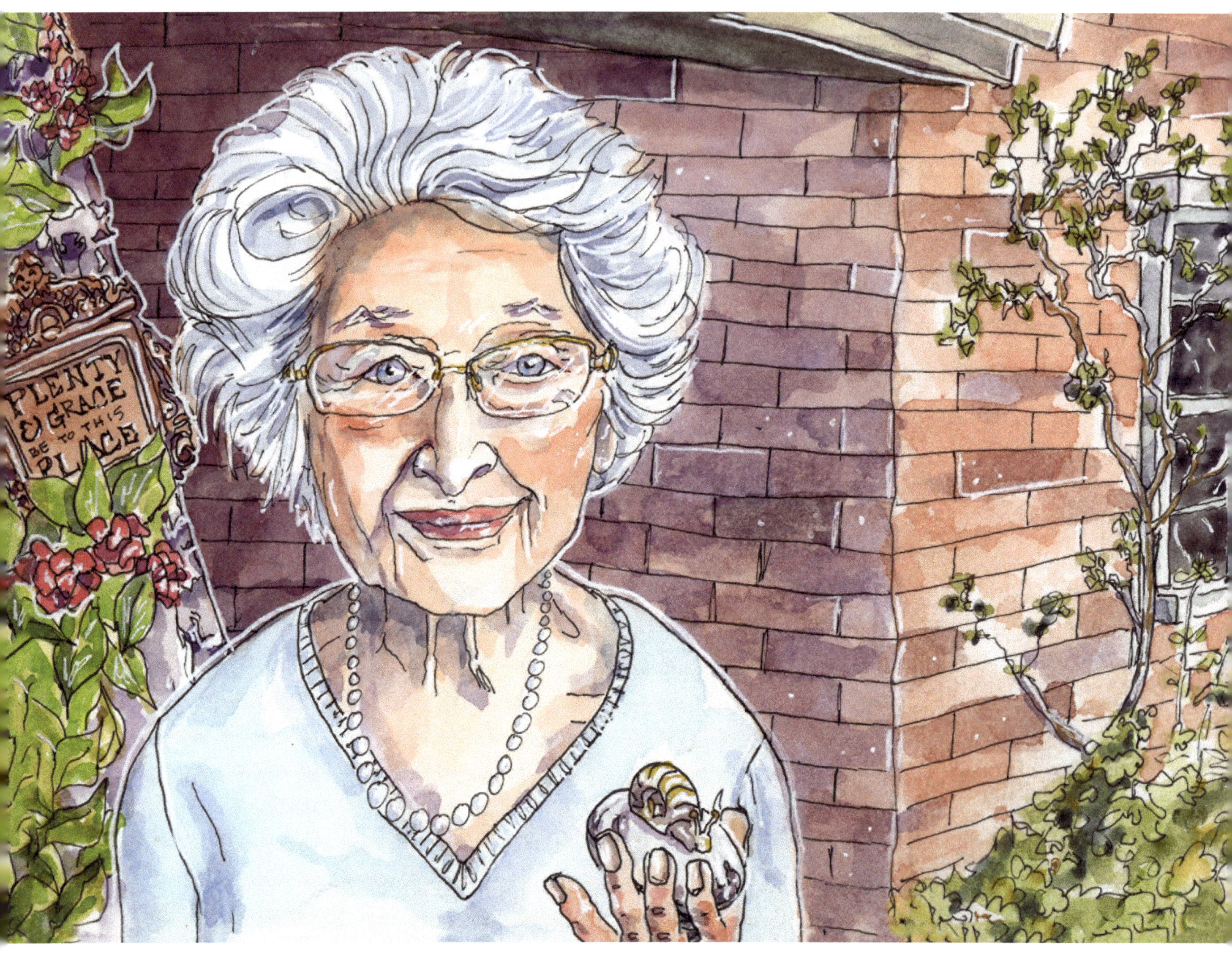
PLENTY
& GRACE
BE TO THIS
PLACE

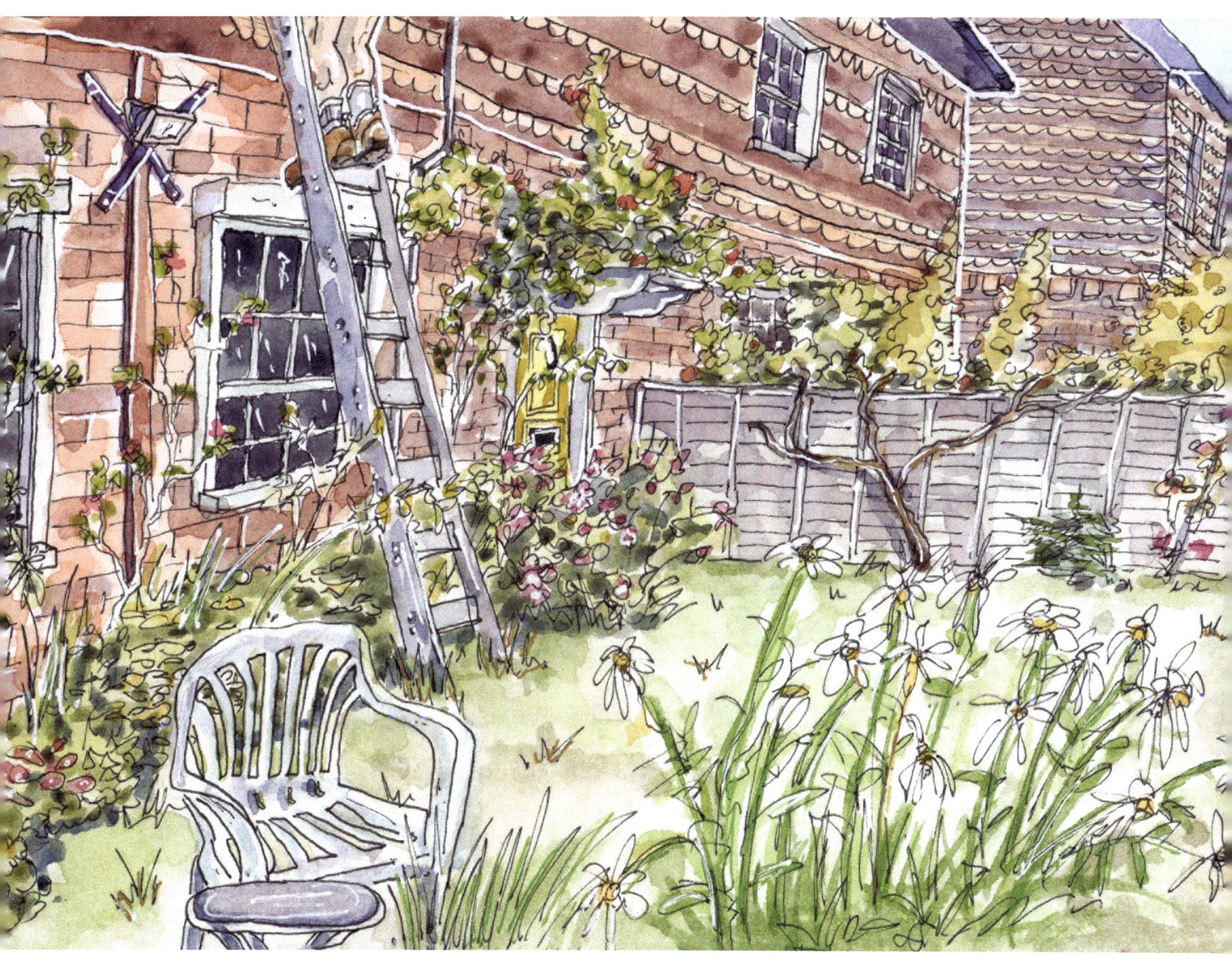

GREAT THINGS DONE

IT WAS MIDMORNING and the temperature had already surpassed an uncomfortable 30 degrees Celsius. My face was radiating an alarming deep crimson glow and the streams of sweat pouring down my brow left my eyes burning from the concentrated saline. After climbing only several hundred feet of altitude, the valley below had fallen away to reveal a hazy veil. Pausing for a rest on a boulder, my climbing buddy and I sloshed down a glut of water and took a few deep breaths. I felt a sharp pang in my chest. This was definitely not the sort of thing I wanted to feel on a remote goat's trail on the side of a rather imposing mountain, in a foreign country without mobile phone service.

The hidden state of my heart continuously plays on my mind; I wonder if, despite all the rest, exercise and medicine, my body is back to fighting form? Naturally, I don't often talk about this for fear of worrying others or, by some irrational self-fulfilling prophecy, giving cause for another heart failure, but it has become an enormous metaphorical mountain in my life. So, in that moment, rather than say anything, I took another swig of water, devoured an energy bar and cracked a joke about my hiking app's poor navigation skills. Then, off again.

My legs were performing well, the muscular endurance that I had built up during my new 'doctor recommended' regime of regular walks and biking had paid off. We clambered up the side of a sharp gulley and emerged from the sheltered col to take on the exposed approach to the summit. Here there was no refuge from the now still, searing heat. Our water stores were perilously low, and I could feel my heart working hard.

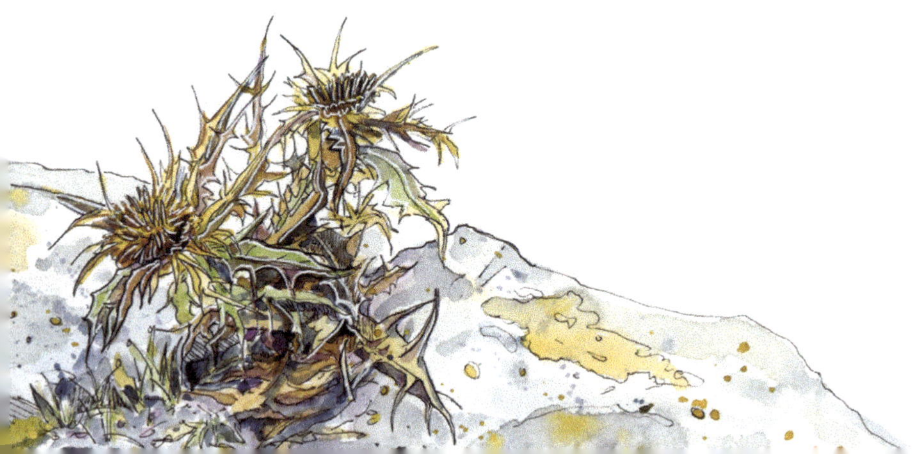

It was at this point, slightly dizzy from the altitude and sun, that I started thinking about how my blood must be thickening up due to dehydration and restricting the delivery of oxygen to my muscles. Again, I silently worried that perhaps this could lead to sinister ill effects on my heart. I carried on, masking the unease with another whimsical quip – now markedly less funny – about thistles and delicate feet.

I have always loved hiking up mountains. Within the journey there is inevitably pain and struggle but there is also thoughtfulness, joy and wonder. William Blake once remarked that, "great things are done when men and mountains meet." Truer words may never have been spoken. I feel that I could walk a thousand foothills but never experience the exhilaration nor depth of revelation as on one mighty mountain.

In another 45 minutes, we had summited, clumsily collapsing by the marker. Reaching into my pocket, I withdrew my phone, and we forced a victorious selfie to mark the accomplishment. Then, with legs dangling over the precipice, the whole world stretching out before us, I realised that I was very much alive, heart beating peacefully in my chest. My body and all the work of the prior months had done their job. A coy smile crept across my face. Then, leaning over to my comrade, I mused, "I can heartly believe we made it. I thought it would be all in vein!"

That day great things were done; I had met my mountain.

*In the Picture: Puig Tomir, Serra de Tramuntana, Mallorca

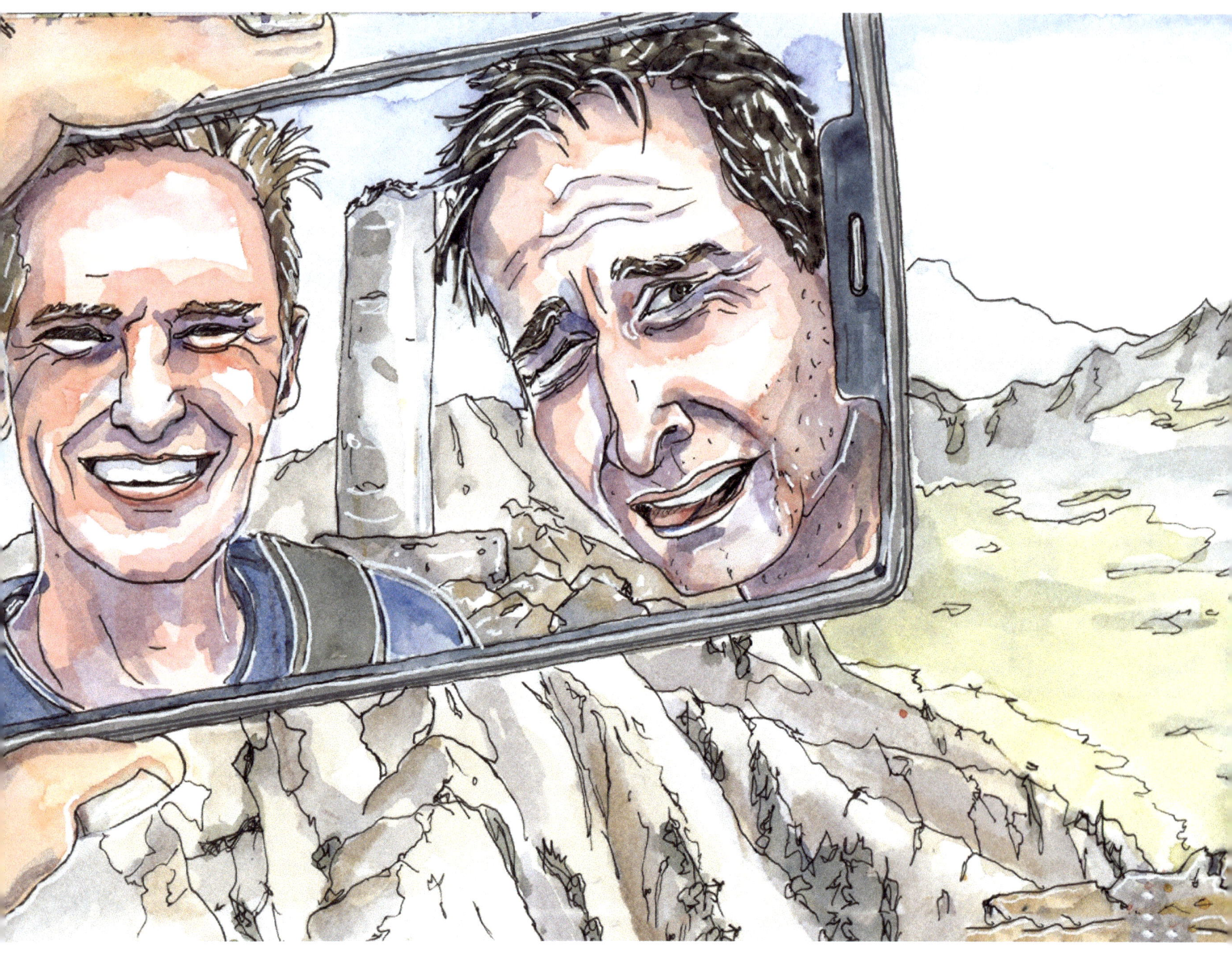

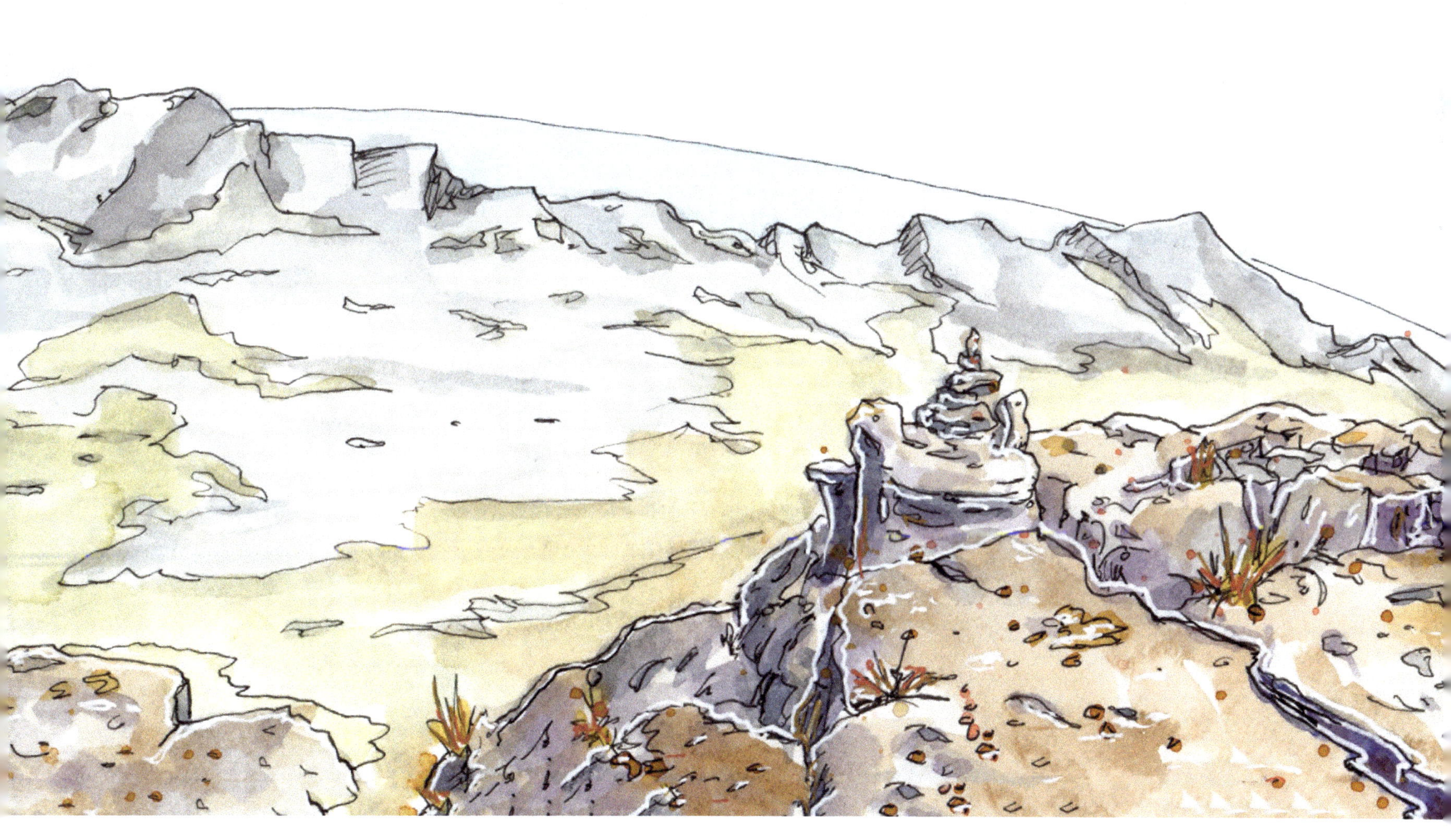

LOOKING UP

WE spend a great deal of our lives looking down, while at work, walking along the street, peering at our devices, eating dinner or just getting lost in our thoughts. Caught in our little delectable worlds, processing life, we often lose sight of the bigger picture.

One fine morning as I vacantly strolled up the quaint street leading to my work, I paused at a local street-side coffee establishment. It was early, so the usual bustle had not yet started. A chirpy young barista took my order and began her artisan process, carefully measuring out the coffee beans. As I stood on the pavement waiting, I impulsively reached into my pocket and slid out my phone. Instantly the screen leapt to life with its whizzy display of colour, but before I had the chance to catch up on the latest news, I was pulled away from that hypnotic moment when the server, in her effortless south London accent, exclaimed, "Gaw, look at the sun on that spire!"

I clumsily looked up, and responded with an uncertain, "What?"

She smiled, pointed and repeated herself, "Look up, sir. Look at the sun shinin' off that spire! How nice is that!"

She was absolutely right. The morning sun had just emerged above the Victorian terracing to illuminate the spire of an old church building, which, coincidently, happened to house the school in which I worked. Staring at the spectacular scene, I ashamedly realised that in my eight years of working at the school, I had never actually taken the time to look up and really examine the intricacies of the building, never mind when it was gilded in warm morning light. In that moment, there was an incredible feeling of calm and joy and inspiration.

This phenomenon is not new. Great minds have been pointing us heavenward for millennia, encouraging us to look beyond our own circumstances and to see the world, the greater context in which we live. When we do this there is a sense of story, one that we all share.

In a recent expedition into London, I popped over to the V&A Museum. It really is a marvellous place, with its collection of rare antiquities and treasures. However, there is a breath-taking moment when you round the corner and enter the central Cast Courts. Sitting within the cavernous hall is a replica of Rome's 200-metre-tall Trajan's Column. You can't help but look up and marvel at this epic monument with its relief frieze telling the story of humanity, its struggles and its victories. I left that day, as I had the little coffee stand, feeling inspired. Inspired to look up more often, beyond myself and savour my place in a greater story.

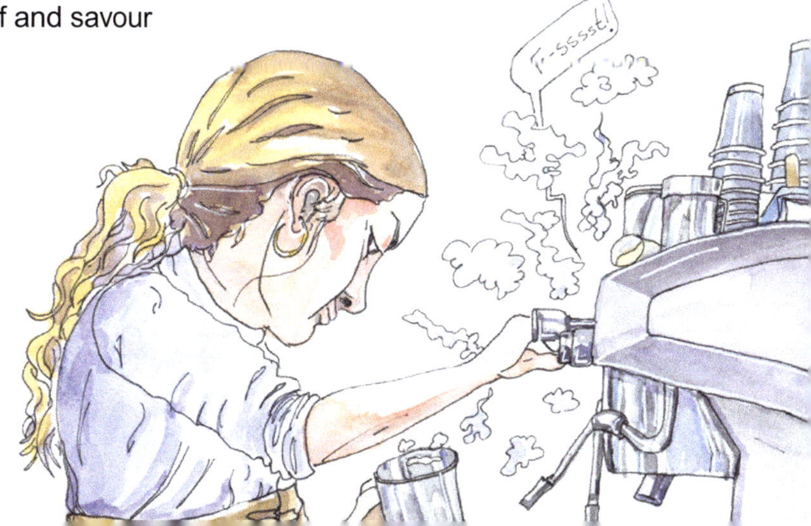

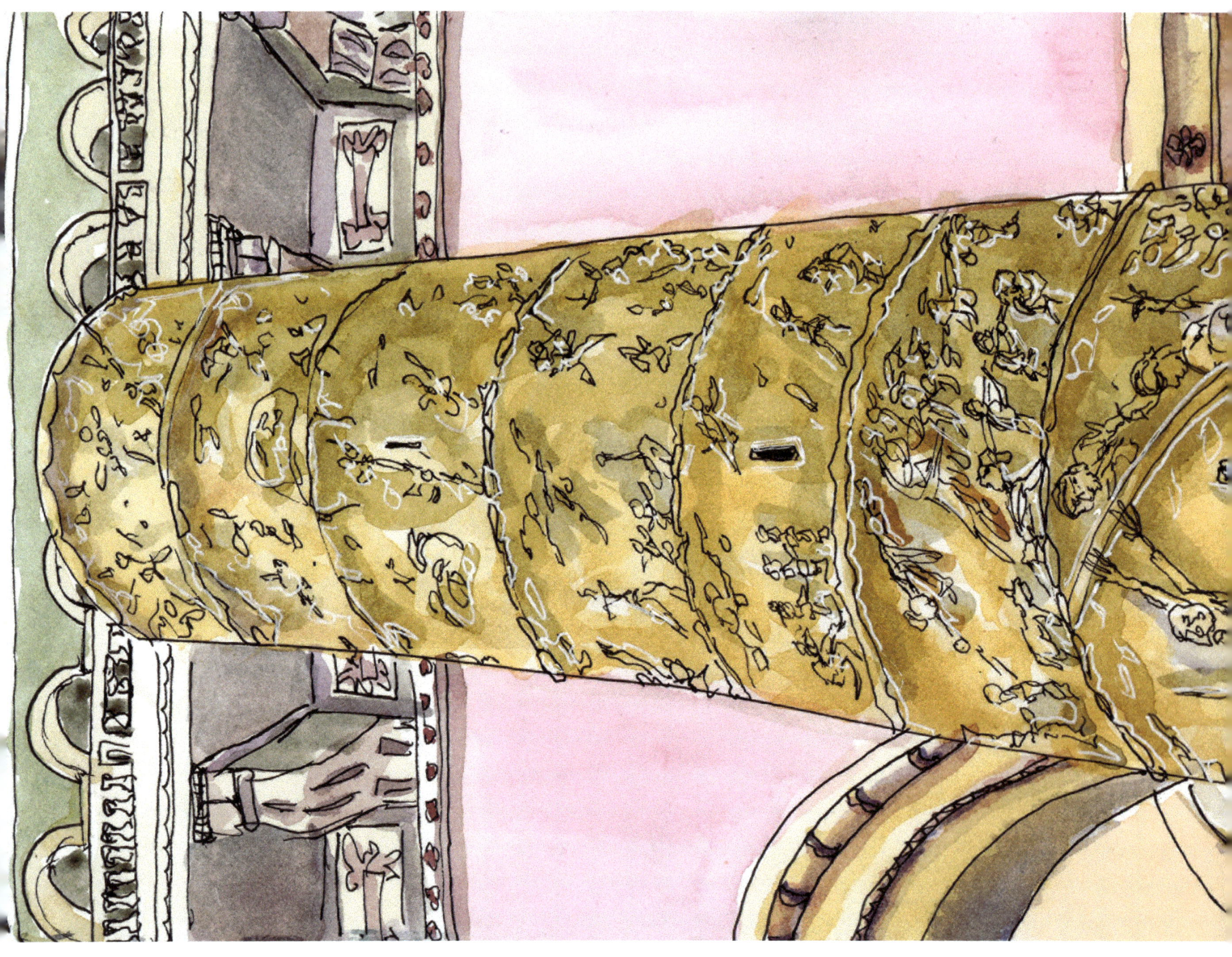

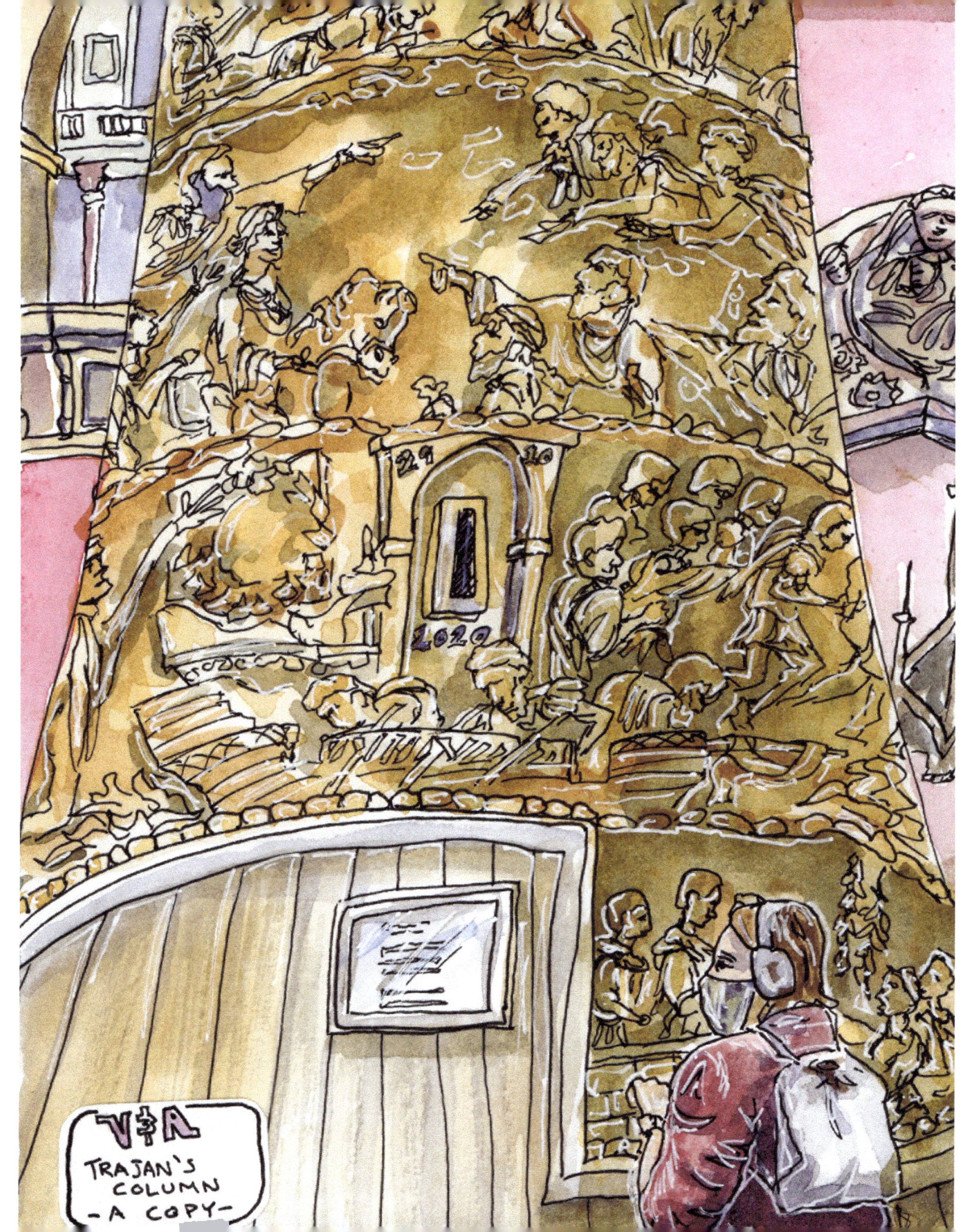

V&A
TRAJAN'S
COLUMN
-A COPY-

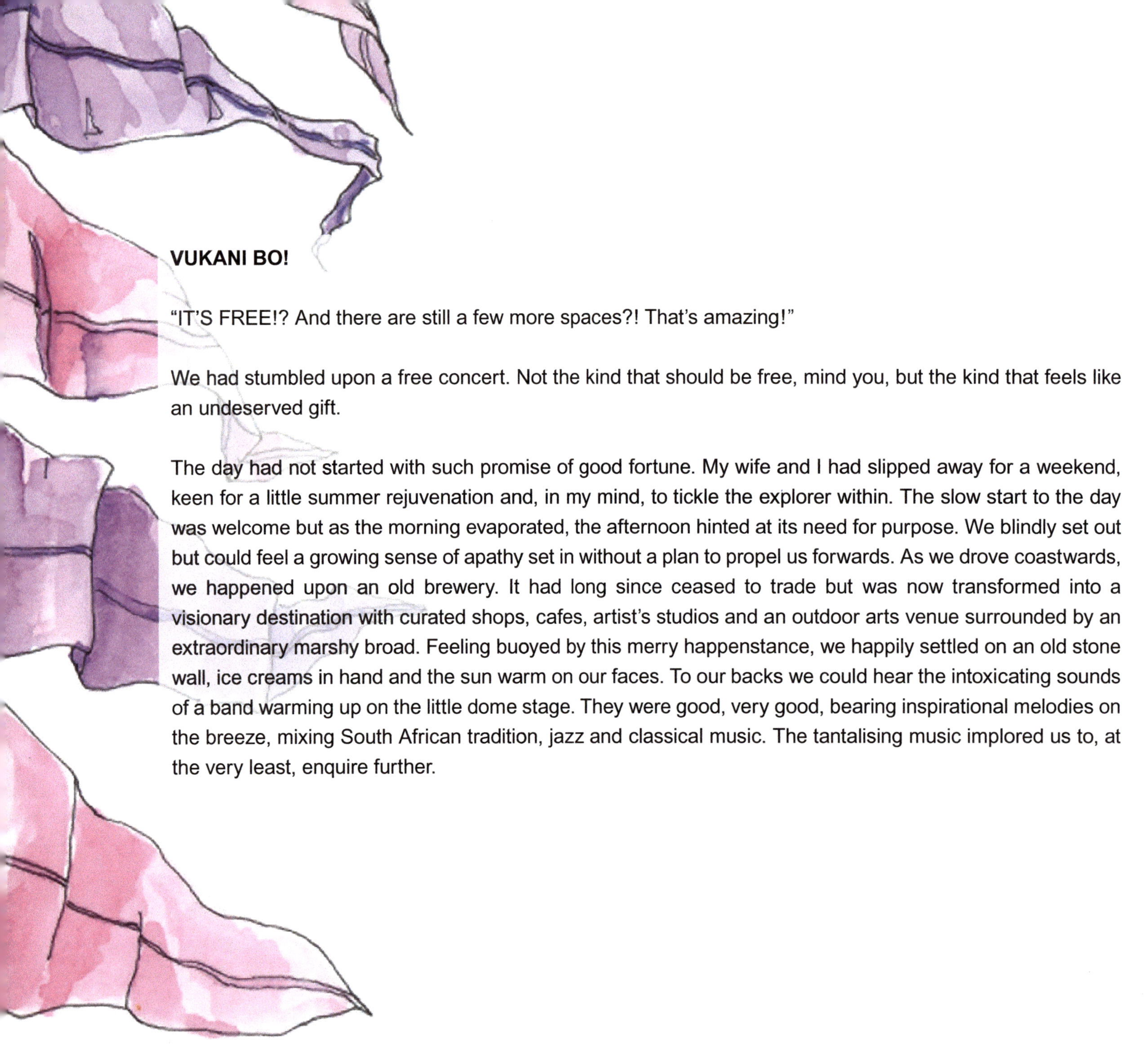

VUKANI BO!

"IT'S FREE!? And there are still a few more spaces?! That's amazing!"

We had stumbled upon a free concert. Not the kind that should be free, mind you, but the kind that feels like an undeserved gift.

The day had not started with such promise of good fortune. My wife and I had slipped away for a weekend, keen for a little summer rejuvenation and, in my mind, to tickle the explorer within. The slow start to the day was welcome but as the morning evaporated, the afternoon hinted at its need for purpose. We blindly set out but could feel a growing sense of apathy set in without a plan to propel us forwards. As we drove coastwards, we happened upon an old brewery. It had long since ceased to trade but was now transformed into a visionary destination with curated shops, cafes, artist's studios and an outdoor arts venue surrounded by an extraordinary marshy broad. Feeling buoyed by this merry happenstance, we happily settled on an old stone wall, ice creams in hand and the sun warm on our faces. To our backs we could hear the intoxicating sounds of a band warming up on the little dome stage. They were good, very good, bearing inspirational melodies on the breeze, mixing South African tradition, jazz and classical music. The tantalising music implored us to, at the very least, enquire further.

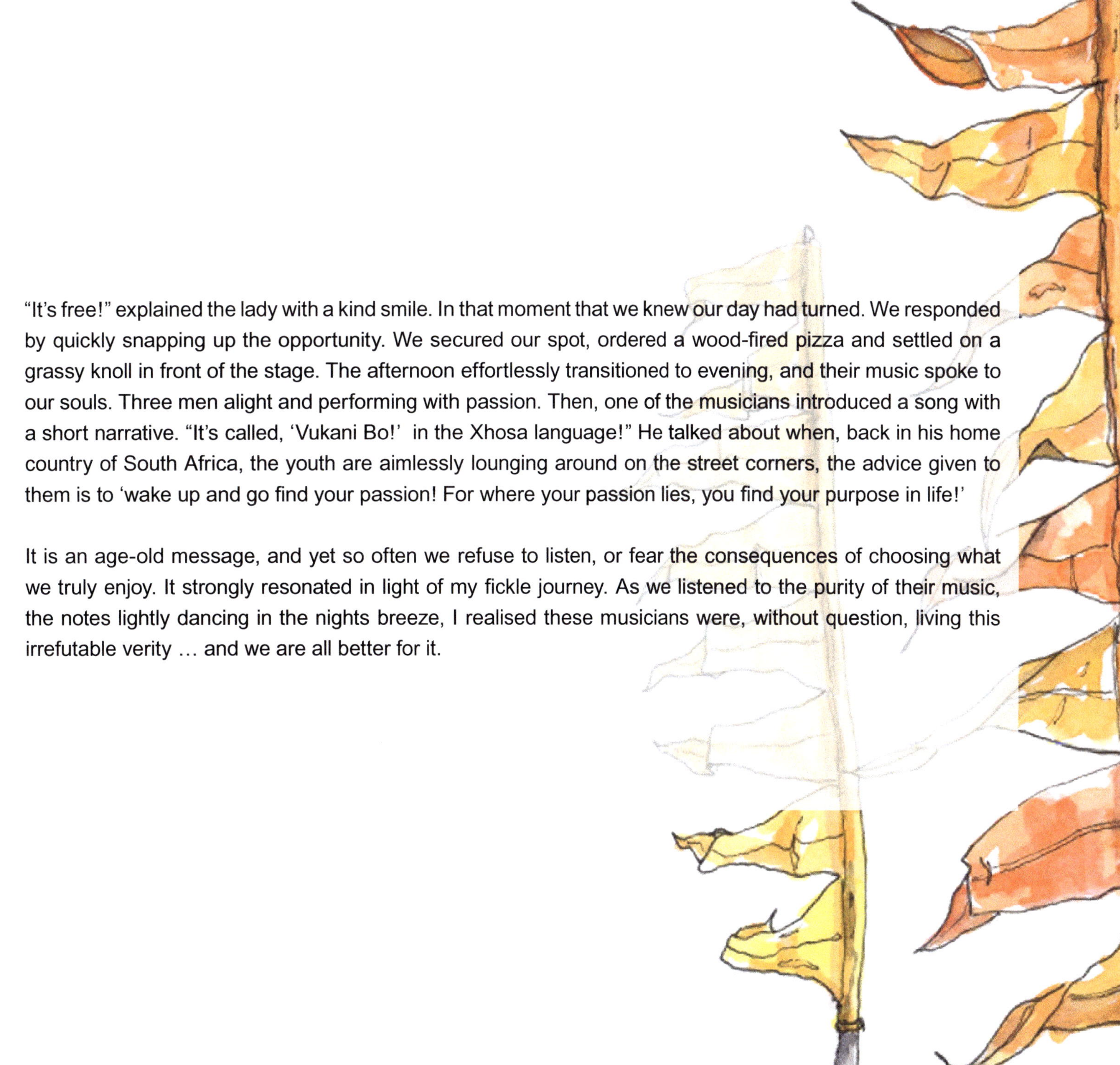

"It's free!" explained the lady with a kind smile. In that moment that we knew our day had turned. We responded by quickly snapping up the opportunity. We secured our spot, ordered a wood-fired pizza and settled on a grassy knoll in front of the stage. The afternoon effortlessly transitioned to evening, and their music spoke to our souls. Three men alight and performing with passion. Then, one of the musicians introduced a song with a short narrative. "It's called, 'Vukani Bo!' in the Xhosa language!" He talked about when, back in his home country of South Africa, the youth are aimlessly lounging around on the street corners, the advice given to them is to 'wake up and go find your passion! For where your passion lies, you find your purpose in life!'

It is an age-old message, and yet so often we refuse to listen, or fear the consequences of choosing what we truly enjoy. It strongly resonated in light of my fickle journey. As we listened to the purity of their music, the notes lightly dancing in the nights breeze, I realised these musicians were, without question, living this irrefutable verity … and we are all better for it.

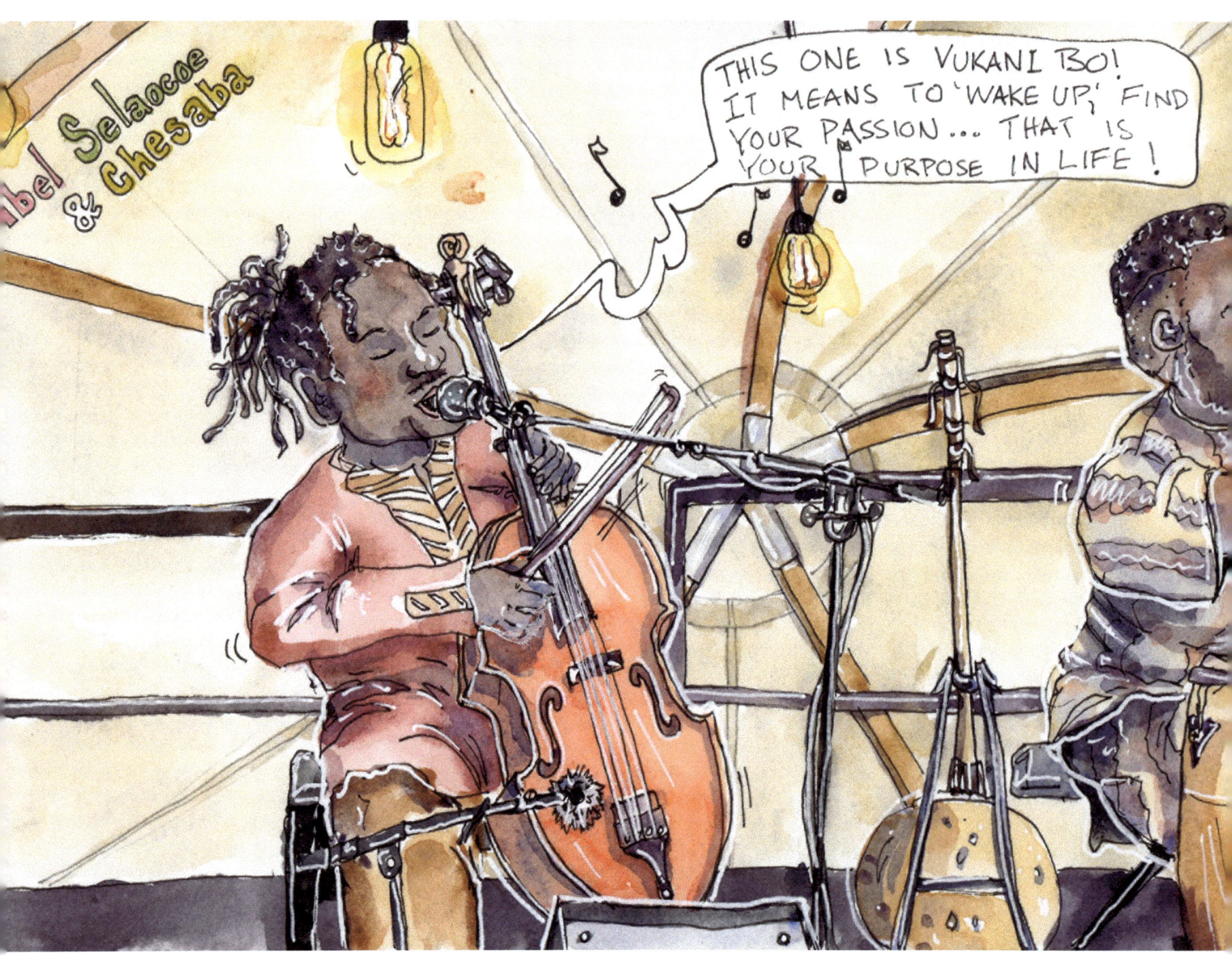
Selaocoe & Chesaba
THIS ONE IS VUKANI BO!
IT MEANS TO 'WAKE UP', FIND
YOUR PASSION ... THAT IS
YOUR PURPOSE IN LIFE !

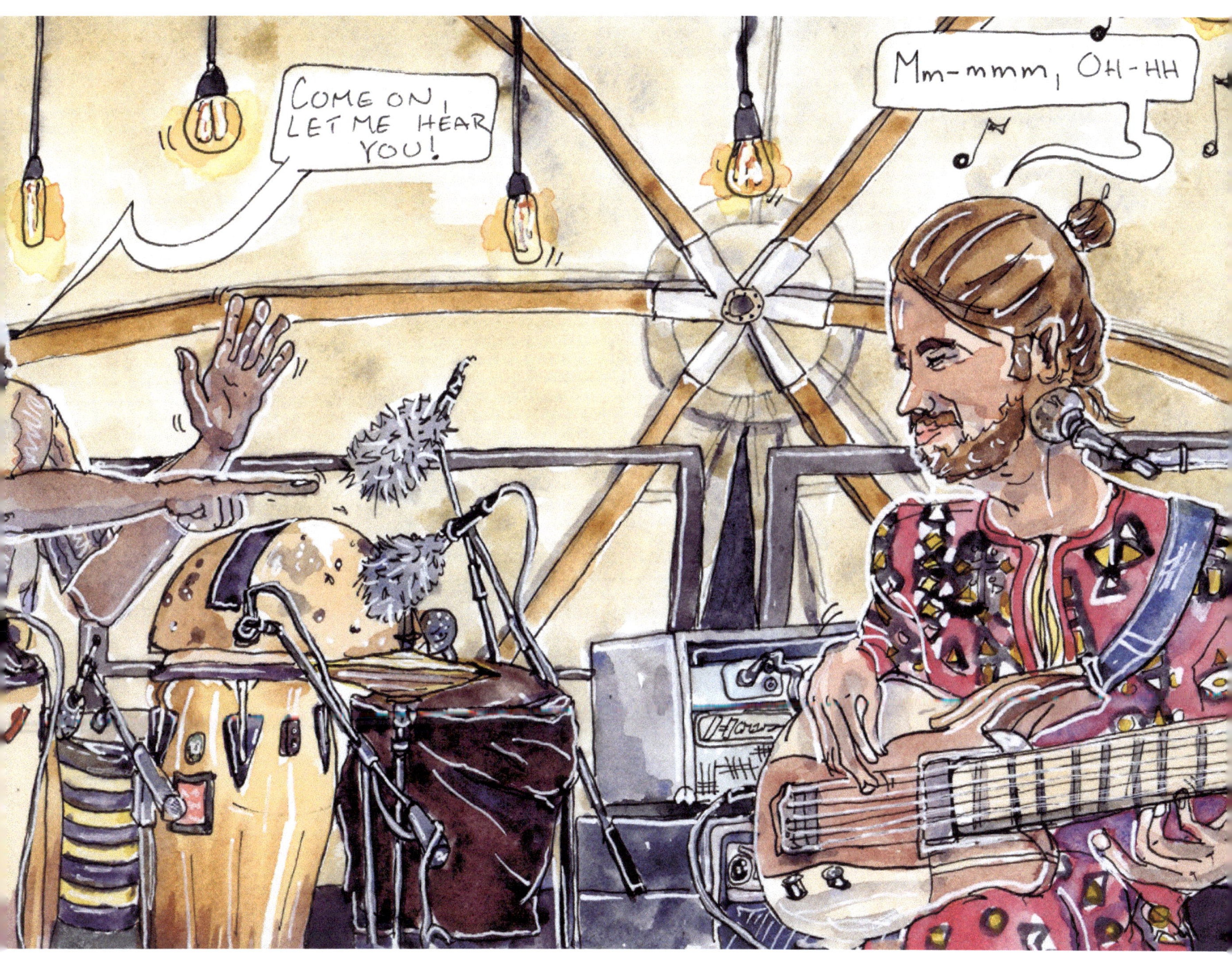
COME ON,
LET ME HEAR
YOU!
Mm-mmm, OH-HH

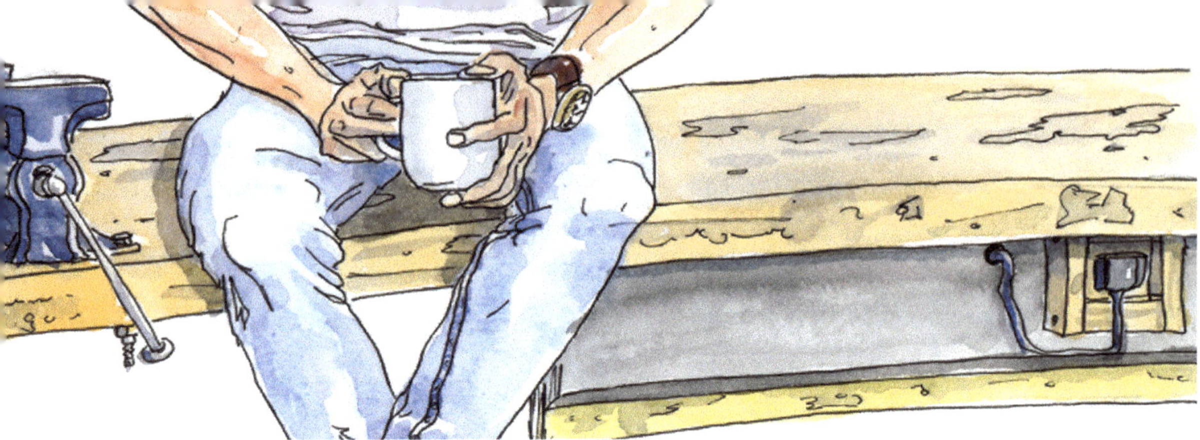

FINDING WHITE SPACE

MOST GOOD THINGS in life begin with a single idea. Sometimes these ideas flow effortlessly, like an elixir from the gods, usually announcing themselves in an unexpected moment of carefree joy. However, all too often, these sparks of genius are elusive, and few and far between. Squeezed into the margins of life, they live in the seemingly unreachable chasms between work, projects, family and fatigue.

I was recently involved in a rather grand theatre project wherein the set required a magical forest. The agreed concept was simple. It would play on the metaphorical layers of story using a series of silhouetted trees clad in fairy-tale script. Each gnarled tree was designed, then programmed into a whizzy CNC machine. The precisely cut trees emerged from the ply revealing their striking form. The offcuts, usually discarded (and disregarded), piled up awaiting disposal. Then, in a moment of downtime, while jovially reclining, legs hanging loosely from a workbench, a friend looked at the pile of 'waste' and noted that the negative space was quite powerful, even beautiful. "Why not use it?" he declared. And so, in that pause, unexpected genius arrived, and a notably more powerful stage-set was born.

This was a marvellous moment of two concepts colliding – the physical reflecting the metaphorical. The value in the off-cut negative space was only unearthed in a period of time when cut away from the task. The negative space was not 'negative' at all. It had become a useful tool, even the star of the show! In design circles this space around a drawing or text is known as 'white space'. It allows the viewer to breathe and fully absorb the content. Like most things in life, space provides an opportunity to see things anew, often with enhanced richness. The view from the top of a mountain, for instance, enables you to see the full majesty of an ancient range, rather than merely the gritty, cumbersome stones that led you up the weathered track. The white space allows you to focus on what is there, what is possible, often hidden in plain sight, and in surprising detail and colour.

The key to this goodness is in finding 'white space', intentional moments within a day to breathe, without assignment. Letting the mind wander free. To step away. To imagine. To create. Think a dog in a park, off its lead, without boundaries. Even the smallest gaps of space can give the oxygen needed to fuel the wildfire of creativity. And possibility. And ideas.

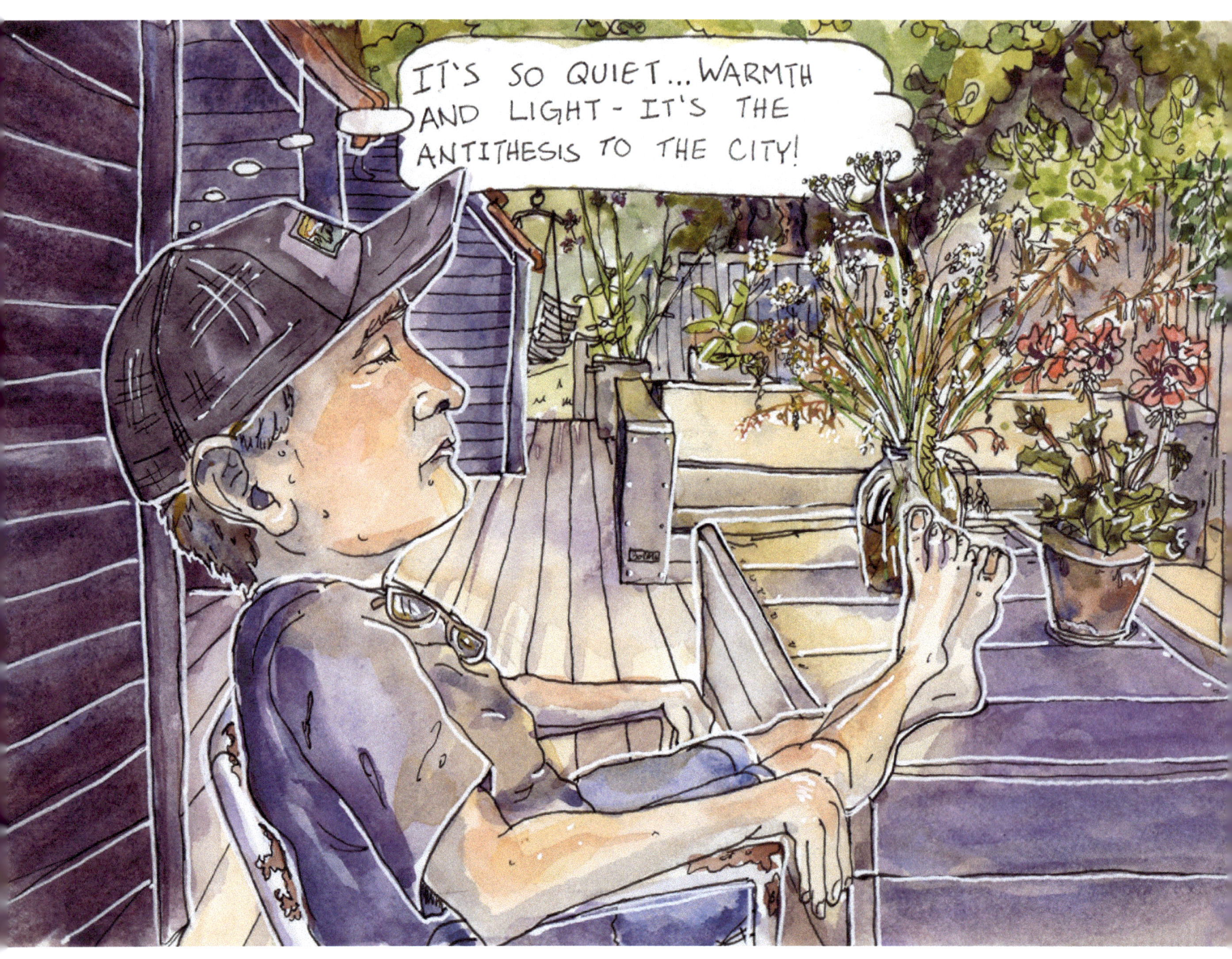

IT'S SO QUIET...WARMTH
AND LIGHT - IT'S THE
ANTITHESIS TO THE CITY!

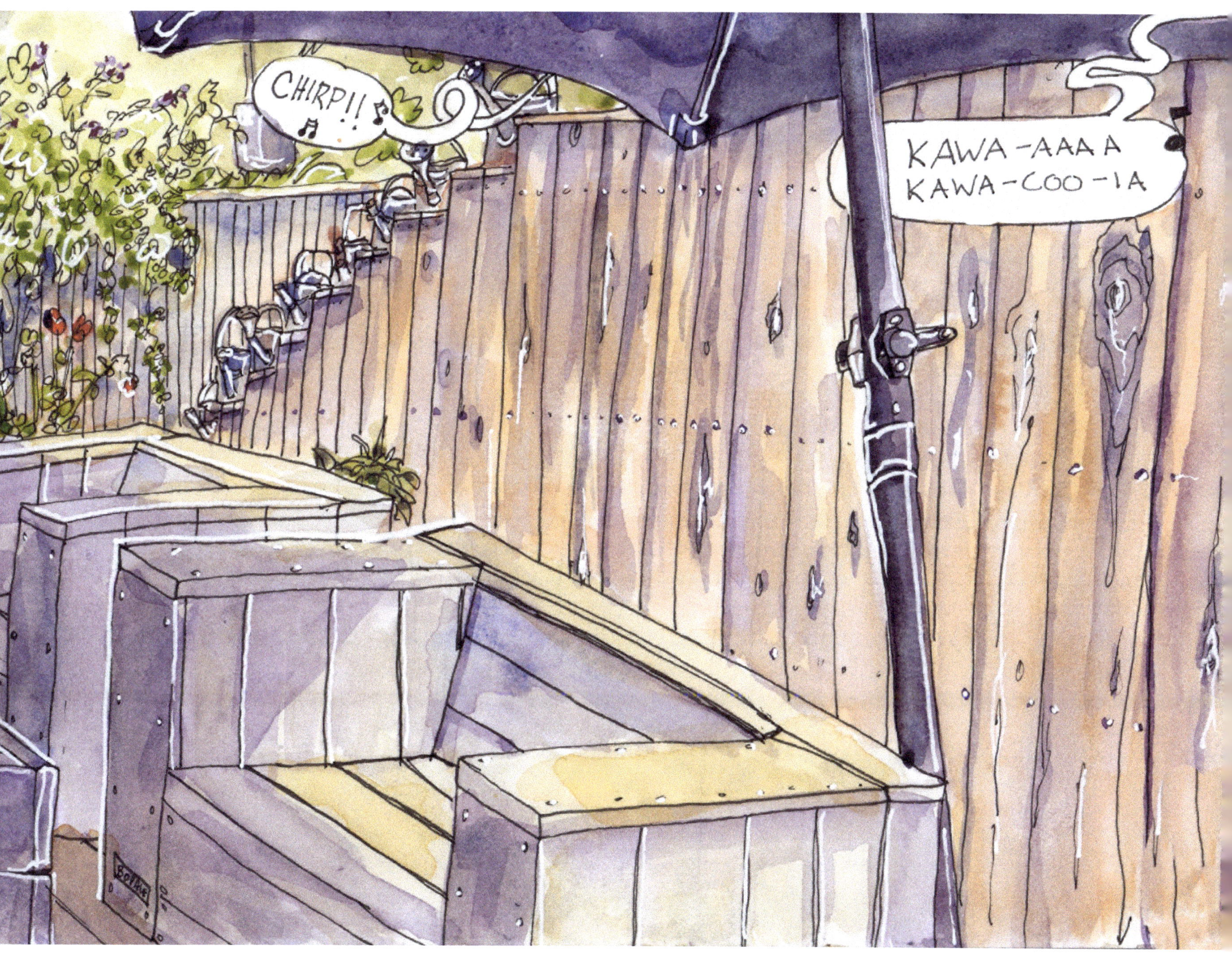

CHIRP!!
KAWA-AAA A
KAWA-COO-IA

A 'HRMPH' AND A 'FULLER' FUTURE

JUST as life seemed to be falling into a neat little package (complete with good health, renewed resolve and an optimistic plan for the future), I had a follow-up conversation with my consultant. In the discussion, and to my surprise, he casually used a rather malicious phrase to describe the condition of my heart, "Let's talk about your 'heart disease'." Despite the trauma of past few months, I had not at all considered that I had a disease. As far as I was concerned, I had simply had a temporary setback. I have spent so much time on the recovery trail, ultra-alert to the circumstances around me and making positive changes that I had missed the fact that there was an underling illness, lying in wait like a thief, to rob me of life when I least expected it.

The doctor continued his probing, "And how are you finding your medication?" Another punch in the gut. Medication has continued to be a constant reminder, twice daily, that I am not the man I was. Defiantly, I responded by explaining that I was feeling tip-top (which was largely true) and then asked a question of my own, "When will I be able to drop some of these drugs?"

He let out a little I've-heard-this-before "Hrmph", then gently duelled back, "My job is twofold: First, it is to keep you alive, and second, it is to keep you feeling comfortable. Both of those things we are successfully doing for you right now."

Touché. - I exhaled my own (defeated) "Hrmph."

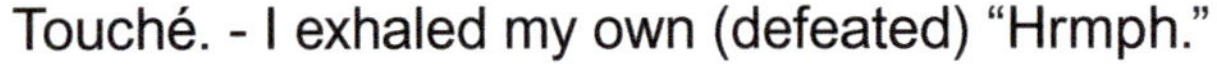

As I reflected on our mano-a-mano, I felt grateful to be alive and keenly aware of how hopeful I am. Then I remembered another recent conversation, this one was with a leading educator. He had shared a parable, of sorts. Traditionally, in indigenous communities, when a plant is sick, they will examine and attend to the environment surrounding it rather than the plant itself, for it is often the environment that is the problem and not the patient.

To a large degree, our immediate environment is one thing we do have control over. Not only can we orchestrate what goes into our bodies, how we rest, work and play, how we interact with others, and ourselves, but we can also choose the future we will step into.

Buckminster Fuller, architect, engineer, inventor, philosopher, author, futurist, teacher, poet and generally talented chap, once said, "You never change things by fighting the existing reality. To change something, build a new model that makes the existing model obsolete."

So, here I am, engineering a new, more tantalising model for my life, with the great hope of positive change. With creativity activated and plans unfolding, my heart feels good, very good indeed.

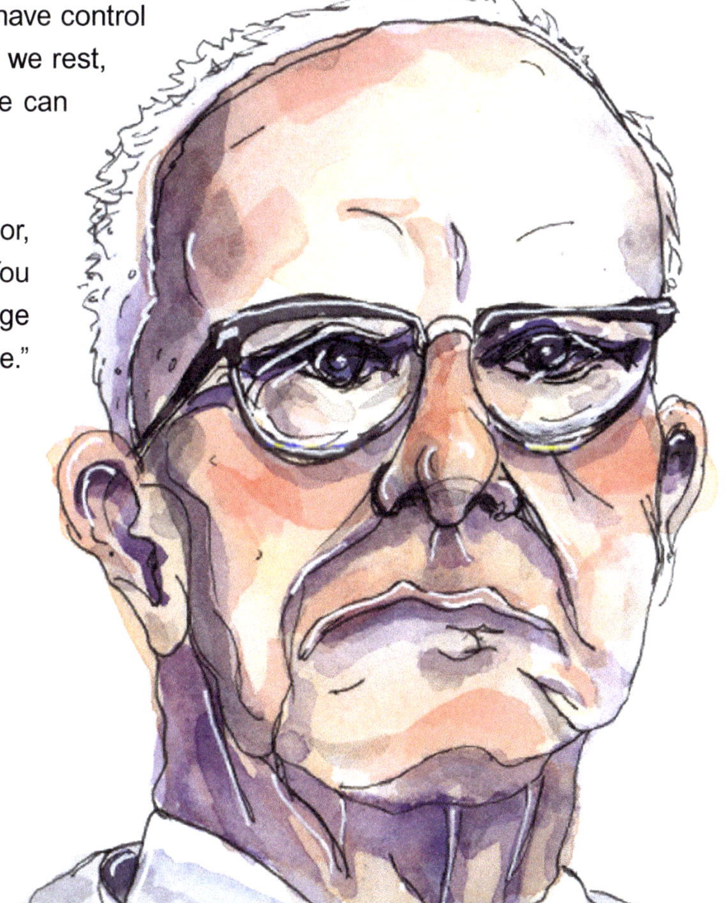

THE WHOLE OF THE MOON

I AM SURE that inextinguishable hope is the key to not only surviving but thriving. I am also pretty sure that, if it were not for hope, my heart would have given up ages ago.

Anne Frank, caught in a seemingly hopeless situation, once said, "What a wonderful thought it is that some of the best days of our lives haven't even happened yet." The ability to wake up and feel that the day ahead might possibly be better than the last is quite a remarkable quality — especially in the face of adversity. People with this outlook exist all around us, sometimes subtly but always effortlessly. They are inspiring and implore us to press onwards. They seem to wear their hope with remarkable ease.

Recently, I had the privilege of witnessing a craftsman of hope in action. I had popped into town one evening after work. It was an unusually warm evening, the old cobbles illuminated by the soft glow of the mock Victorian streetlights. There were people about, the restaurants and cafes full of revellers enjoying the final embers of summer. And there was music. At first, I thought it was coming from within one of the buildings, but the sounds were too vibrant to have been contained behind walls. "A concert," I thought with delight! (I love music and the joy that it brings. I think there must be a special place in heaven for musicians.) Peering down the pedestrianised street I saw no sign of any performers, but the music was very much there and alive. I veered off my intended route to try to discover where this ethereal delight was coming from. Then, halfway down the hill, I spotted a figure reclining on a bench, the light of a nearby shop highlighting his rough contour. I drew closer, he was clearly a gentleman of simple means. He had a well-used trolley neatly packed with treasures and a little red ghetto blaster perched on his tummy from which he was unapologetically blasting his music.

His head swung down over the edge of the bench, and he flashed me a wide (nearly) toothless grin, then continued to croon the verse of a song, harmonising perfectly with the tape player. I recognised the tune that was dancing through the night air, the classic 80s rock beat and distinctive vocals unlocking memories from my youth. With unabandoned passion he continued belting out the old Waterboys hit.

I spoke about wings
You just flew
I wondered, I guessed and I tried
You just knew
I sighed
But you swooned, I saw the crescent
You saw the whole of the moon
The whole of the moon

It was as if he saw something I didn't, the wholeness of life, and I, only fragments.
I watched with wonder. He warmly glanced at me, winked, then turned his gaze heavenward and continued singing. Here was a man, bearing all the marks of a life scared with trauma yet not allowing those circumstances to dampen his resolve. He sang with conviction and of possibility. I wandered off, smiling, my mind feeling the prospect of infinite possibilities ...
... perhaps that is what hope is, the ability to dwell in possibility.

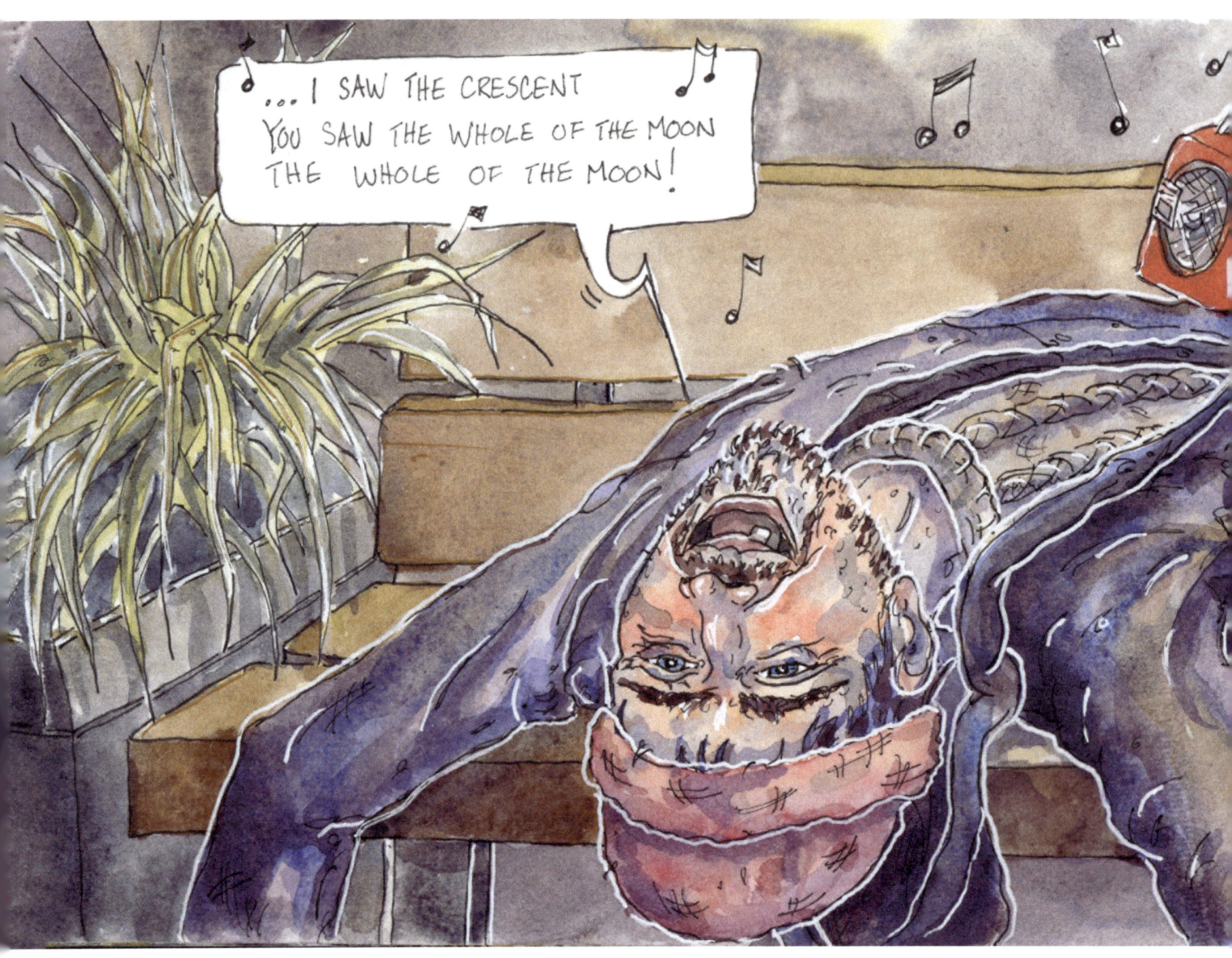

...I SAW THE CRESCENT
YOU SAW THE WHOLE OF THE MOON
THE WHOLE OF THE MOON!

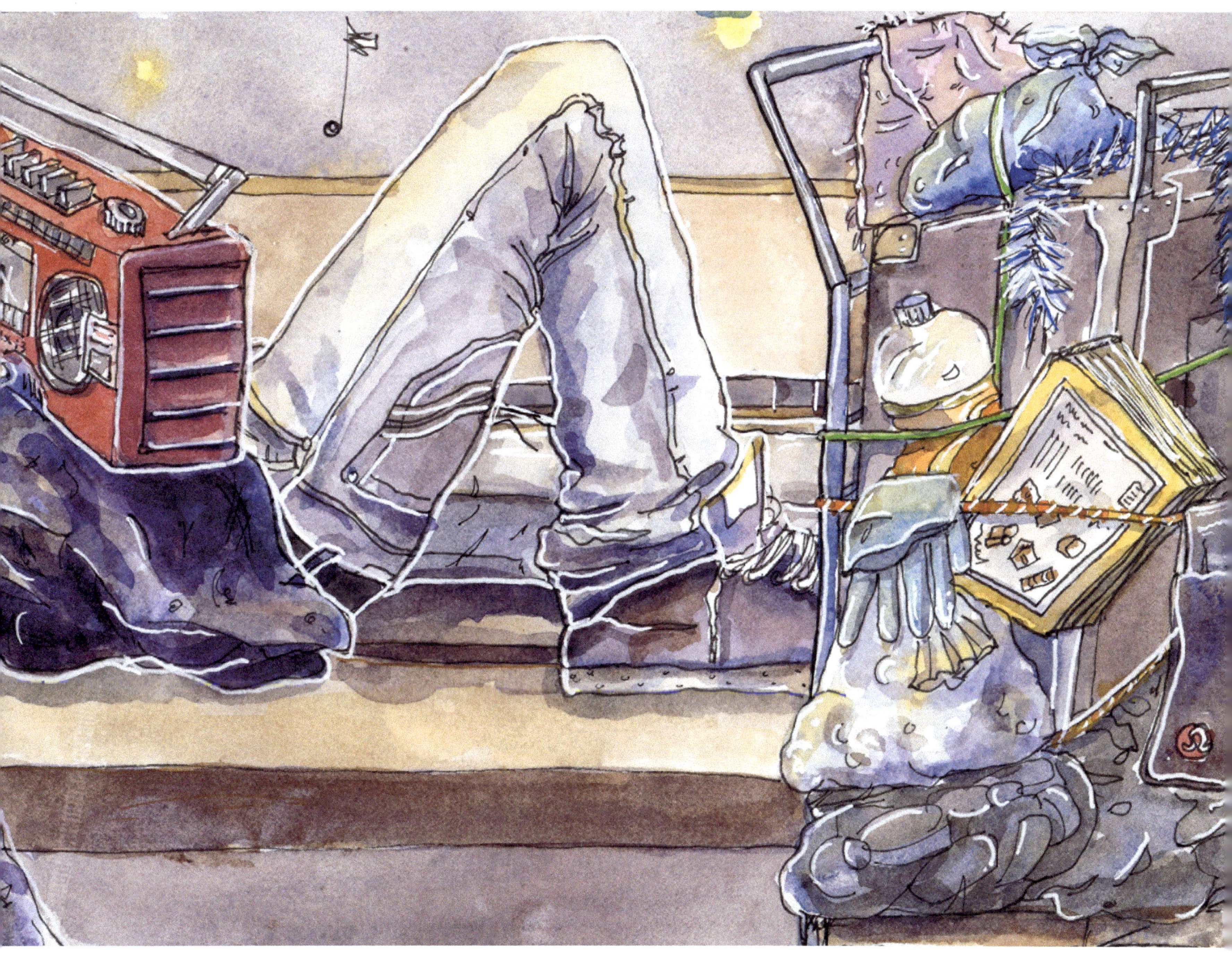

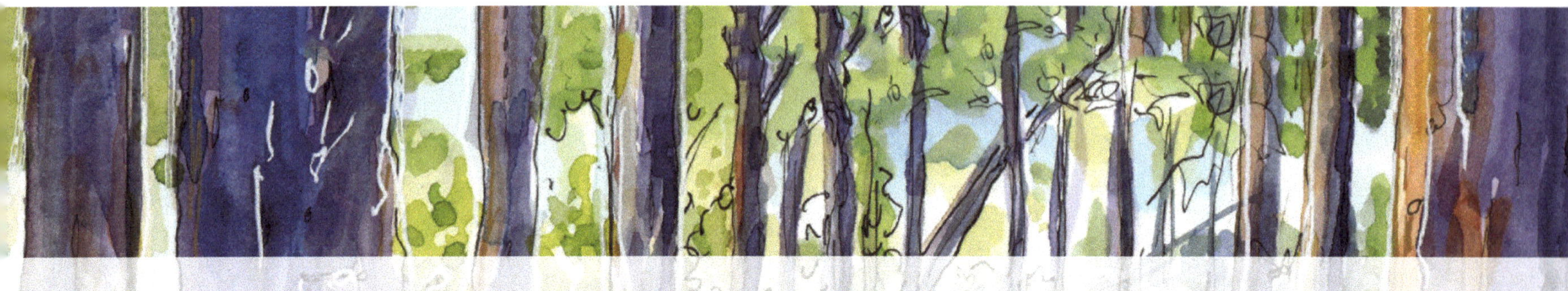

NOT JUST A STATISTIC

ACCORDING to statistics*, 7.6 million people are living with heart and circulatory diseases in the UK. These cardiac ailments account for a quarter of all deaths. That's roughly one every three minutes! Staggering! These statistics are, quite literally, not for the faint-hearted.

Thankfully, we are not defined by numbers. They create part of the context of our life, but they certainly don't define us. When I started this journey, I could not see past my immediate circumstances and most certainly could not foresee an optimistic outcome. In those days, hope was rare, like that of the sparsely dappled light on a forest floor. It was an uncertain time and all-consuming. I felt I had failed in my journey to live a rich, epicurean life and, worse, I was scarred by trauma – another statistic. However, now, after ticking off nearly a year on this journey, and having made significant changes, there is a sense of renewal, beams of warm, rejuvenating light colouring the world around me.

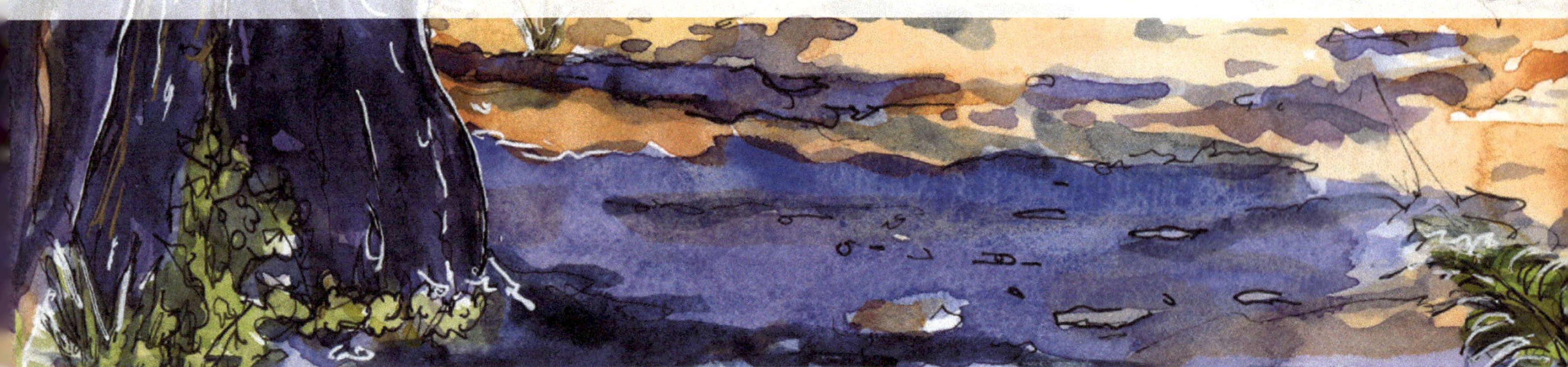

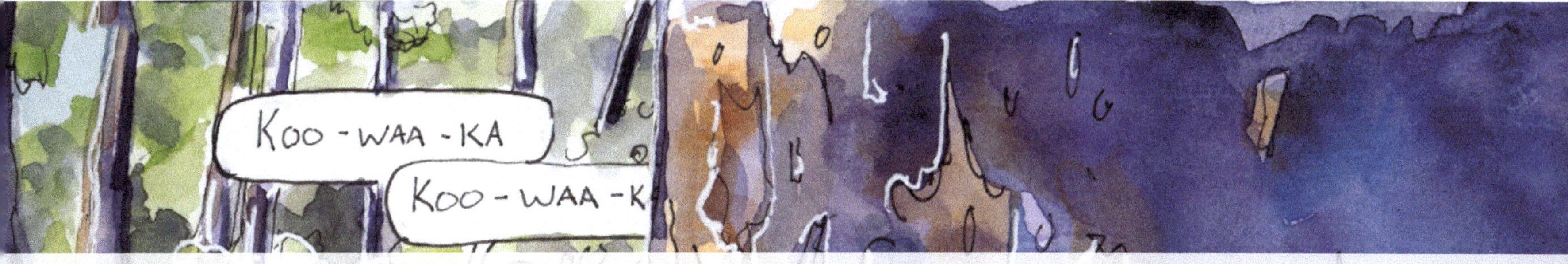

Light really is an extraordinary thing. It can cut through the darkest shadows and illuminate the most amazing details. On an evening walk along a particularly dramatic stretch of Cornish coastline, I marvelled at the high untamed cliffs. They had taken endless beatings from the restless ocean yet still they stood their ground. As the sun lowered on the horizon, I watched in awe as the warm light dissolved the shadows formed by rocky crags and, as I climbed the tumbled boulders, I began to notice extraordinary nuances, marvellous details that I had not seen before. A damp residue on the stones served to enhance the rich multitude of colours – iridescent blues, mysterious purples, deep ochres and rich reds! These colours, seen from afar, were lost in the vast story of time. But in that one precious moment, it was clear that at the heart of every journey, every life, there is a vibrant patchwork of unique experiences that make up a rich and beautiful story ...

... a 1 in 7.6 million story.

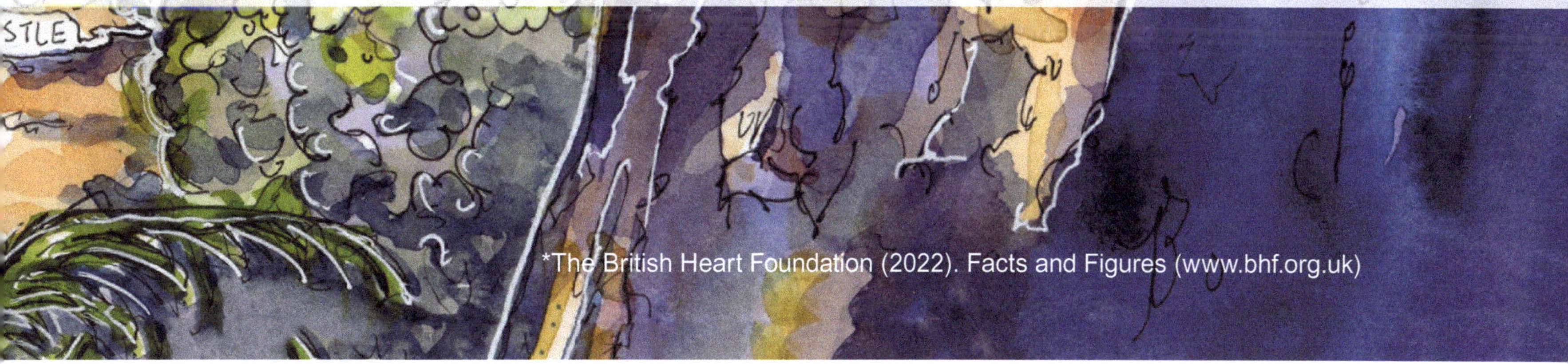

*The British Heart Foundation (2022). Facts and Figures (www.bhf.org.uk)

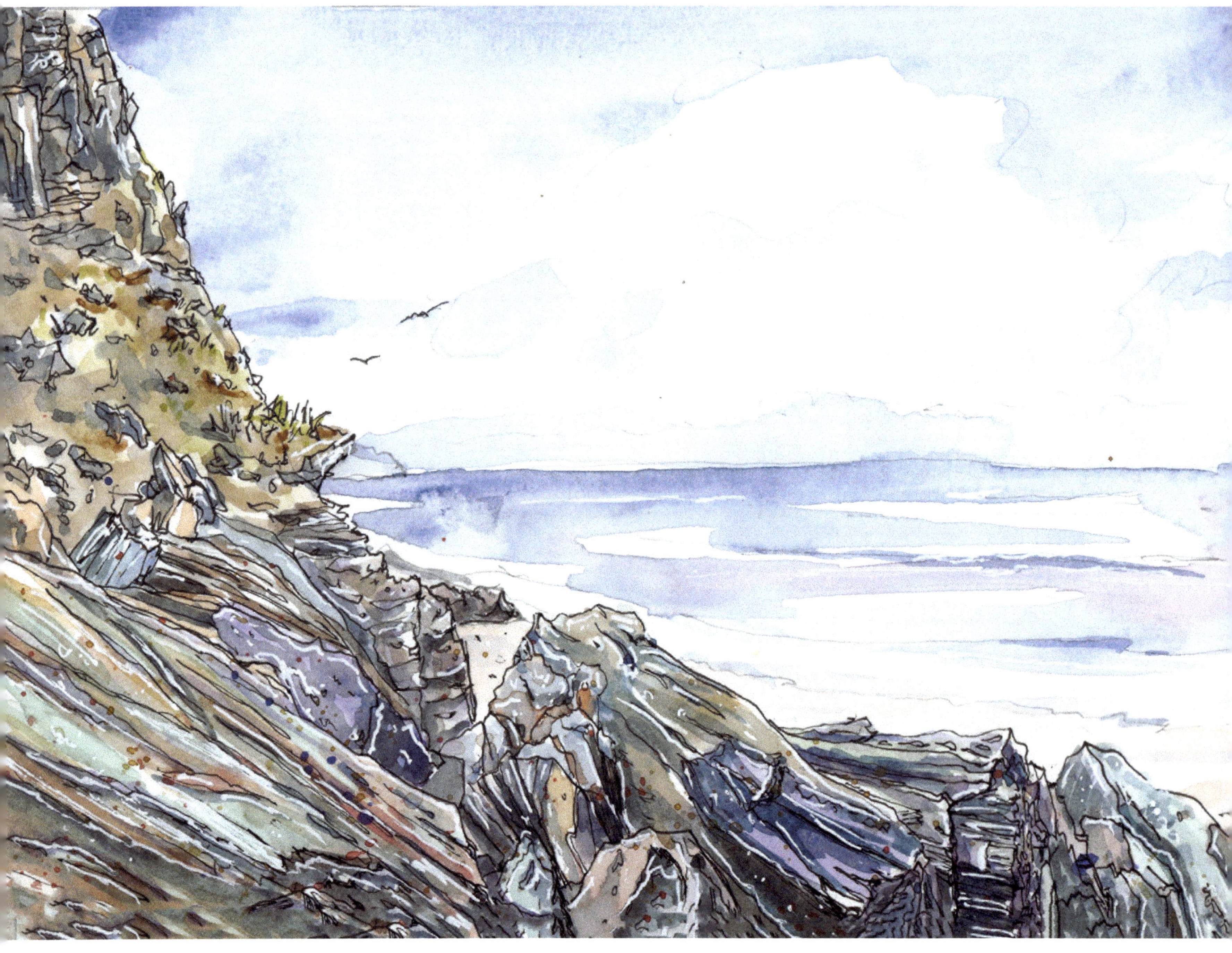

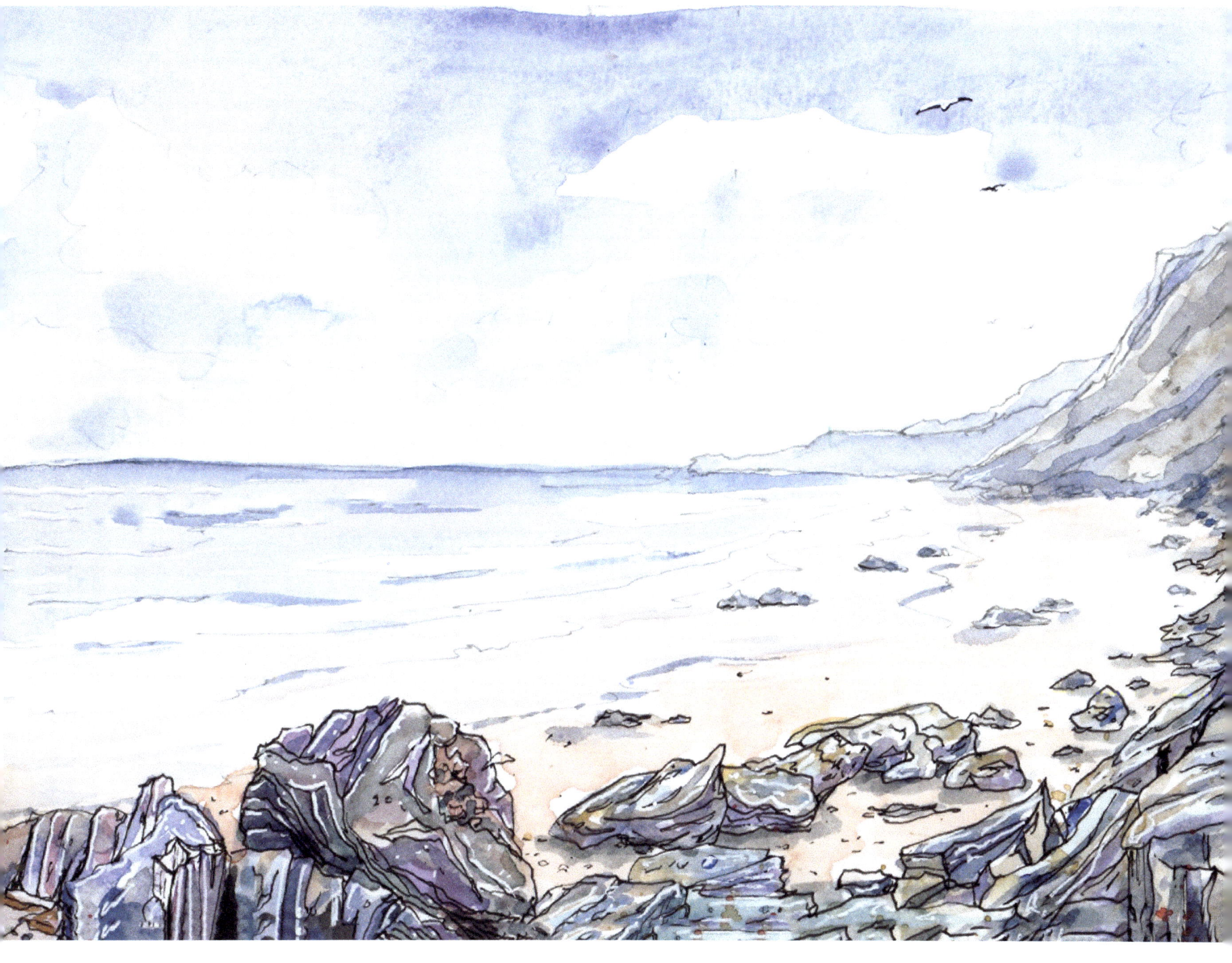

PS. LIVE INSPIRED

AFTER PRECISELY ONE YEAR of cold toes and unnatural bruising, I was happy to celebrate this first birthday with a return to St Georges Hospital for a review and an echocardiogram. Although this time my mode of transport was slightly less fluorescent-light-gilded coach, I arrived, as I had a year earlier, in a state of fluster. I had been held up by several construction blockages and the Friday school run traffic, and so I found myself sprinting to make my appointment. With my heart wildly pounding in my chest, I feared I might have a repeat cardiac crisis. But despite my underlying worries, I slid through the doors of the specialist wing with a minute to spare. I smiled. A year ago, this run could have killed me, but now, as I sat in the waiting-room chair, heart rate neatly falling, I felt satisfied that all was well.

It wasn't long before I was called by Tíana, a young Irish sonographer, who performed the echo with grace and ease. Naturally, I am now much more interested in the workings of the heart and so, as she probed my chest, I asked an abundance of questions. I was surprised to hear that at that moment there were roughly 150,000 other people in the Greater London area awaiting that same test! Unbelievable! Heart disease is a very real issue for so many people. It affects each in their own way. For some the outcome is understandably scary, while others use it as a springboard to flourish.

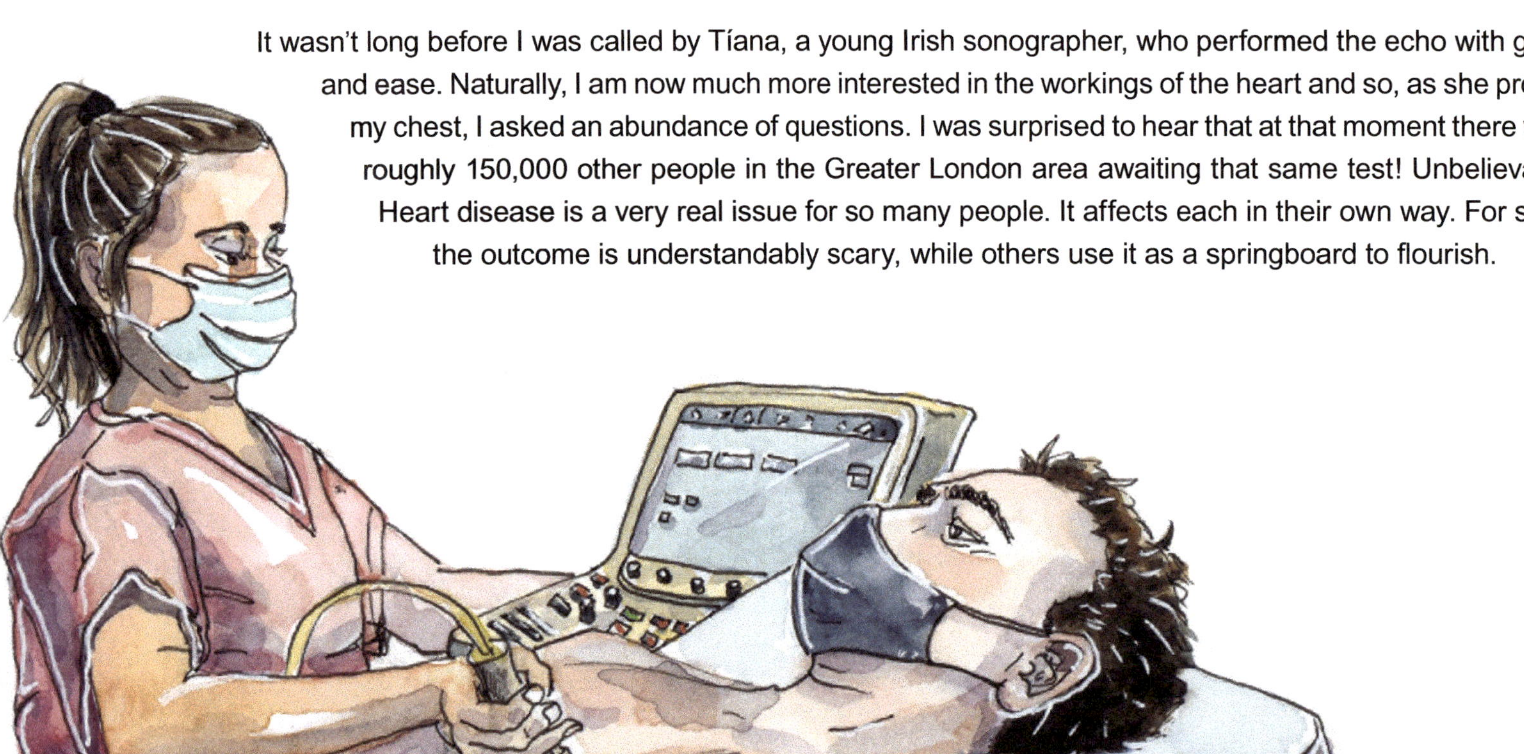

So, how are the others in this book fairing a year on?

- Mark is now doing well. Impressively, he stopped smoking 'cold turkey' on the day that he entered hospital a year ago. He noted that it was "a shame it took a heart attack to give them up." He continues to look forward, making changes that will enable him to reduce his current regime of heart medications.
- David too has embraced a new improved life. Despite five stents and two heart attacks, he is still led by compassion, has completed the entirety of Hadrian's 80-mile wall on foot and has embraced a wholesome diet enhanced by his wife's spicy kimchee!
- Sadly, during the writing of this book, the tentacles of heart disease have reached even the most inspiring of individuals – Jean. In mid-Autumn, Jean suffered a series of heart attacks. Upon hearing the news, I went to visit her. She was noticeably frailer, but despite a panic button now mounted on her left wrist, her eyes still twinkled as she spoke of hope. Determined to keep her ticker going, she is daily completing six robust circuits of her garden.
- As for me, I still feel occasional palpitations, shortness of breath (perceived or not) and the fear that a heart attack could, at an unexpected moment, strike again. However, despite all of this I feel a deep sense of satisfaction in my new and simpler life. I have also dropped a drug (Ticagrelor) and amazingly, my toes are warmer! I still love to explore, to create, and to look forward.

If I could give just one piece of advice to someone experiencing trauma or adversity, I would say, without reservation, live each day unequivocally inspired.

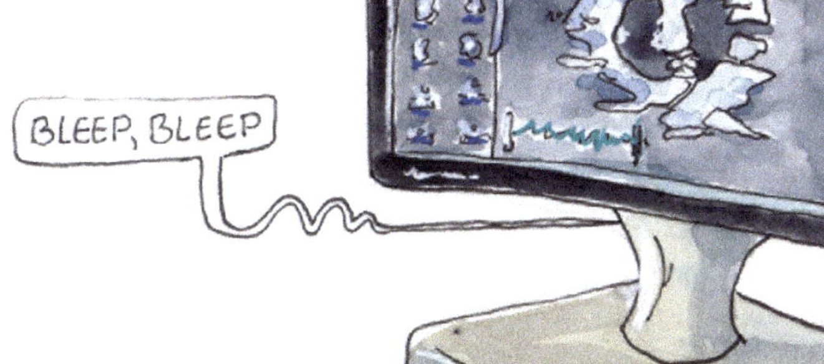

ACKNOWLEDGEMENTS

THANK YOU to my family for sustaining me with love and hope during my recovery and in the time that it took me to write this book – my wife, Anna, for her unflinching belief in me, my daughters, Jael and Jette, for their limitless love (and patience) and Josh for his unerring passion for adventure.

To Esther, Janet and Di I am deeply grateful for the work you have done with the words in this book.

To my marvellous friends who have stuck with me, from trauma through to renewal, I have been infinitely buoyed by your encouragement, insight and cheer.

I am indebted to the many people who have sustained me along the way – in and out of hospital. You have invited me into a life-changing journey and have extended the limits of my understanding of humanity. I am grateful to the artists who have led the way, showing me how to capture the nuanced beauty in this extraordinary world.

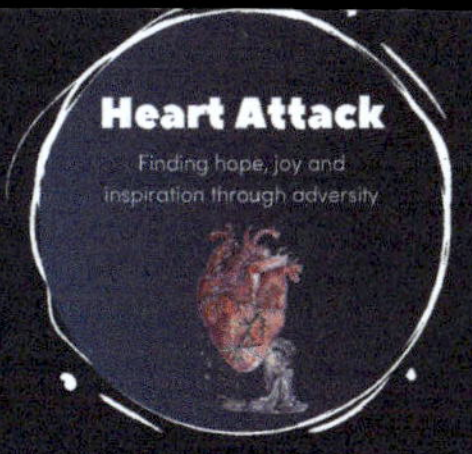

Leave a Review

THANK YOU FOR READING MY BOOK!

I really appreciate all of your feedback. I love hearing what you have to say and your stories of renewal. Your input is so helpful in encouraging others in their journeys through trauma and will improve the quality of resources offered with this book.

Please take two minutes now to leave a helpful review on Amazon letting me know what you thought of the book:

https://subscribepage.io/Review

Live inspired,

Jeff Schmidt

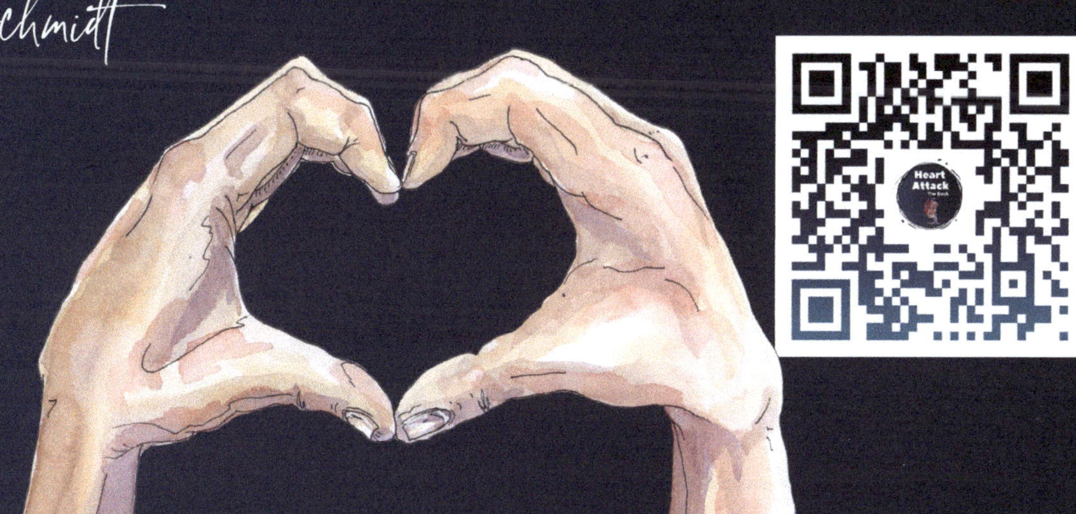

JEFF SCHMIDT is an educator, author,
illustrator, speaker and aficionado of
a life well-lived. Originally from the
tall grass prairies of Canada, he now
lives in the UK with his intrepid wife
and kids. He fills his days inspiring
and being inspired, exploring
the world and documenting its
goodness.

Live Inspired

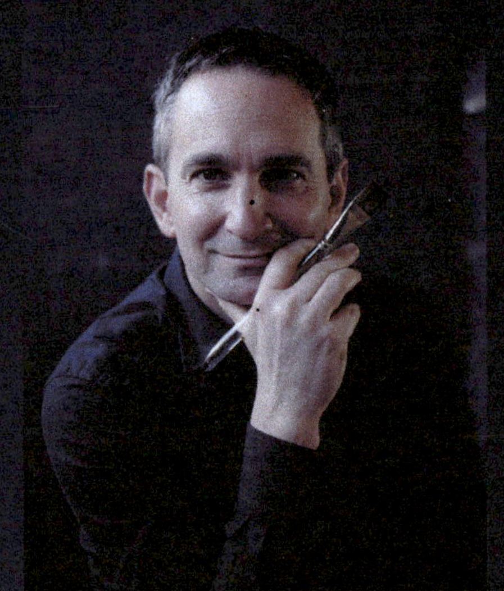

instagram.com/psliveinspired/

facebook.com/psliveinspired/

heartattackthebook.mailerpage.io

Download your Guide Free

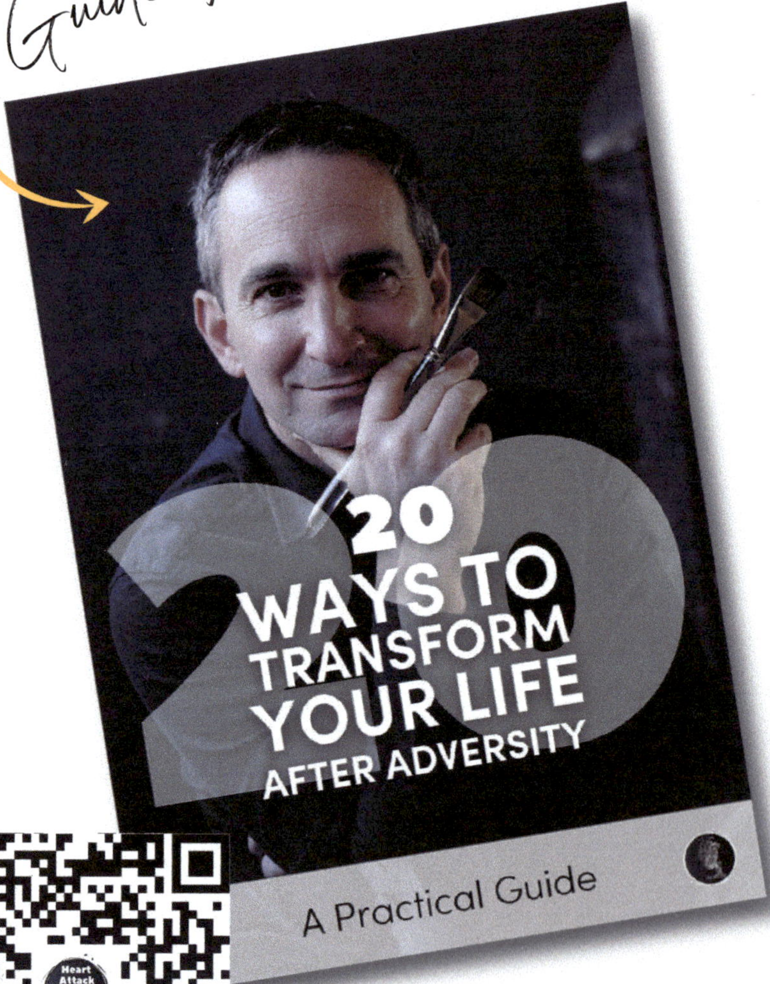

https://heartattackthebook.mailerpage.io